THE TRUTH ABOUT WHIPLASH

A guide to getting better

Chris Connelly, DC

INTRODUCTION

Traffic collisions effect millions of people every year around the world. There are three groups of people after a collision: the people who develop relatively no pain, the people who develop acute pain and the people who develop chronic pain. Approximately 50% of people have relatively no pain and 50% have acute pain. Up to 50% of the people that have acute pain develop chronic pain. With proper management this number can be cut in half. Reducing the number of occupants that progress from acute pain to chronic pain is the goal of this book.

My name is Dr. Chris Connelly and I am a practicing chiropractor in Stone Mountain Georgia. I have been in private practice for over 20 years and have been blessed over this time to have treated over 5000 traffic injury patients, 150,000 chiropractic adjustments, 250 impairment ratings and over 1000 claim reviews for insurance companies. Through clinical practice, reviewing claims of injury and study of current research, I have put together this book for the purpose of getting people better following traffic related injuries.

There are 10 big ideas that I would like to relate to any reader:
- The mechanism of acute pain is not the same as the mechanism of chronic pain.
- Catastrophizing, fear, and worry about pain will actually create the very pain that you fear.
- Tissue damage typically heals in a predictable timeframe. Give the body a chance to heal.
- Pain really is in the mind, but not in the way you think.
- Pain depends less on what is happening in the tissues. Pain depends on what the brain thinks is happening in the tissues.
- Patients with musculoskeletal pain and people without musculoskeletal pain often have similar findings on MRI and x-ray.
- If you hurt your back and get an early MRI, you've reduced your chances of getting better.
- If you think that you will get better, you are halfway to recovery.
- Taking responsibility for your personal health and happiness is not just your duty, but it's your obligation.
- Focus on getting healthy and being happy, not the pain. Make health a habit.

After reading the 10 big ideas for this book some may feel that I have neglected the structural or anatomical components of traffic injuries. I have chosen to cover aspects of healing and pain because other aspects of traffic injuries have been well covered in the following references:

American Medical Association: Guides to the Evaluation of Permanent Impairment, sixth edition. Chicago, American Medical

Whiplash: evidence base for clinical practice, Michele Sterling PhD, Churchill Livingstone, 2011

Whiplash and Mild Traumatic Brain Injury, Arthur C. Croft, Spine Research Institute of Sa; 1st edition (2009)

Whiplash-Associated Diseases, American Medical Association, Rene Cailliet, 2007

Motor Vehicle Collision Injuries, Second Ed, Lawrence Nordhoff, Jones & Bartlett Publishers 2005

ODG Guidelines from Work Loss Data Institute, 2018

The Anatomy & Biomechanics of Acute and Chronic Whiplash Injury, Traffic Injury Prevention 2009, 10: 2, 101-112

This book is divided into 5 chapters: Traffic Collisions, Pain, Vehicle Damage and Occupant Injury, Diagnosis & Tissue Damage and Preventing Chronic Pain. At the beginning of each chapter are quotes that lead into a brief chapter summary followed by the body of the chapter. At the end of each chapter are some definitions to assist with the chapter as well as references for further reading.

More than 100 million Americans struggle with chronic pain, according to one Institute of Medicine estimate, at an annual cost of as much as $635 billion in treatment and lost productivity. Further, the misuse of potent opioid painkillers, meant to help manage pain, can actually increase the risk of addiction, death and pain. We are in the mists of a chronic pain and chronic disease epidemic. Preventing acute pain from progressing to chronic pain is part of the solution to the chronic pain epidemic.

The paradigm shift and core emphasis of this book is to transfer responsibility for your well-being from external factors (doctors, surgeries, medications, testing, therapy) to an internal factor (you). Of course, there are many situations where external remedies and advice are needed, but the way you think and things you do have a significant bearing on your health. You will find that many of the recommendations in this book are also helpful for other pain-related disorders, including work and sports injuries.

Traffic collisions are not just a problem in the United States. Australia, England and Canada have studied traffic injuries extensively and developed guidelines for patient recovery. Some of the materials presented in this book are from these recommendations and guidelines. A few key suggestions from these resources are:

- Those who continue to work, even in a reduced capacity at first, have been shown to have a better recovery than people who take a long-time off work.
- Change the way you do things to reduce strain and pain. Preventing reinjury is a way to recovery.
- Many people recover within a few days or weeks. For others it may take several months to experience substantial improvement in symptoms. Ongoing symptoms may vary in their intensity during the recovery period. This is normal.
- Some people may feel distressed after a traffic collision and these feelings usually settle with time and recovery.
- Managing your thoughts and actions is a key part to stopping the discomfort that you are experiencing.
- Sometimes less treatment, testing and procedures is more effective.
- Invasive procedures intended to "fix" incidental pathologies, that are not the pain generator, are dangerous and harmful.
- Staying active is important.

It is my sincere hope that you find something in this book that prevents progression of acute pain to chronic pain. If you already have chronic pain I hope that you find something that helps to break the chronic pain cycle. It's time to take control of your health and flourish!

My eternal thanks and love go to my wife, kids, family, friends, colleagues, patients, and God, because without them this book would not be.

CHAPTER 1
TRAFFIC COLLISIONS

Most "accidents" are due to negligent driving and are therefore not accidents.
When it happens to you, it's important.
The term "whiplash" should be banished forever.

SUMMARY – Traffic injuries have become an international medicolegal and social dilemma. The highest price we pay for traffic collisions is in the loss of human lives, however society also bears the brunt of the many other costs associated with motor vehicle collisions. According to the National Highway Traffic Safety Administration (NHTSA), traffic collisions are a significant cause of loss of life, productivity, medical costs (short-term and long-term), disability, and property damages.

Millions of collisions occur each year, with most occupants either not being injured or fully recovering from their injuries. Unfortunately, some collisions do result in serious injury, permanent impairment, and even death. Most "accidents" are due to recklessness and human neglence, and therefore are preventable and not accidents. Reducing the number and seriousness of accidents, promoting effective management of injuries, reducing fraud, education, research and public awareness are essential to combat this massive problem.

According to both the US Dept. of Transportation (USDOT) and the National Highway Traffic Safety Administration (NHTSA), traffic accidents can be broken down this way– On average, from year to year, Motor Vehicle Crashes (MVCs) in the U.S. are statistically very similar: Approximately 6,000,000 total reported accidents per year and approximately 3,000,000 claimed injuries per year. Collisions are largely the result of:
1. Impaired drivers
2. Speeding
3. Reckless driving

The majority of patients involved in traffic collisions will recover, but some will have continued symptoms. According to a study from the University of North Carolina School of Medicine, more than 70 percent of occupants injured who visit the emergency room still feel pain 6 weeks later and at 12 weeks, approximately 25% of the injured will still have some symptoms or pain. Traffic injuries are a multifactorial intertwining of social, neurological, psychological, and biological components. Some important predictors of long-term pain following a traffic collision relate to psychosocial factors and aspects of pre-collision health, rather than to various attributes of the collision itself.

INTRODUCTION

In the study of disease, or epidemiology, one of the aims is to assess the risk, the independent association with a disorder, and prognostic or risk factors. To say that the epidemiology "whiplash" is complex is an understatement; even the term "whiplash" is unscientific, flawed, and confusing, but we will address that later. Traffic injuries are very costly on multiple levels, and the problem appears to be getting worse in the US and other nations.

FACTS ABOUT TRAFFIC INJURIES

In America, our favorite and principal method of transportation is by motor vehicle. We drive cars, trucks, SUVs, and motorcycles in cities, towns, and across busy highways to get to work, school, or anywhere else we need to go. With all of this traveling, and the vast number of vehicles on the roads today, it is no wonder that many accidents occur every day. Persistent pain and disability after trauma have become an increasingly significant problem in many industrialized countries, with extensive individual as well as social costs.

The associated and subsequent pain as a result of traffic collisions is a significant health burden for patients and the healthcare system. The escalating costs of injury claims are a concern for everyone. Here we will take a brief look at some facts, figures, myths, and fraud relating to traffic accidents across the U.S. and other parts of the world.

Crashes are one of the foremost causes of death and injury in the world. Motor vehicle crashes are a leading cause of death in the US, with over 100 people dying every day. More than 4 million drivers and passengers were treated in emergency departments as the result of being injured in motor vehicle traffic crashes in 2015. The economic impact is also noteworthy: in a one-year period, the cost just from medical care and productivity losses associated with occupant injuries from motor vehicle traffic collisions exceeded $250 billion.

The National Highway Traffic Safety Administration (NHTSA), a division of the U.S. Department of Transportation (DOT) that was established by the Highway Safety Act of 1970, works to reduce and prevent the ill-effects of traffic accidents, including injuries, deaths, and economic losses. The NHTSA uses statistics to analyze the success of safety programs and to determine what areas need the most attention. The following statistics have been compiled from information offered by the NHTSA:

National Statistics show that:
- The National Highway Traffic Safety Administration estimates about 10 million or more crashes go unreported each year.
- In 2016 there were 6,296,000 police-reported motor vehicle traffic crashes; 37,461 people died and 2,443,000 people were injured. An average of 96 people died each day in motor vehicle crashes – one fatality every 15 minutes.
- Private insurers pay approximately 50% of all motor vehicle crash costs. Individual crash victims pay about 26%, while third parties such as uninvolved motorists delayed in traffic, charities and health care providers pay about 14%. Federal revenues account for 6%, while state and local municipalities pick up about 3%. Overall, those not directly involved in crashes pay for nearly three-quarters of all crash costs, primarily through insurance premiums, taxes and travel delay.
- More than half (51 percent) of people killed in car accidents in 2010 were not wearing a seatbelt at the time of the crash.
- New findings from the Insurance Research Council's (IRC) Auto Injury Insurance Claims Study shows that medical expenses reported by auto injury claimants continue to increase faster than the rate of inflation, in spite of the fact that the severity of the injuries themselves remain on a downward trend.
- Nearly half of all fatal crashes occurred on roads with posted speed limits of 55 mph or higher.
- In 2016, 10,497 people were killed in alcohol-impaired driving crashes (any fatal crash involving a driver with a blood-alcohol content (BAC) of 0.08 percent or higher), up 1.7 percent from 10,320 in 2015. Of the persons who were killed in traffic crashes in 2016, 28% died in alcohol-impaired driving crashes.
- Motor vehicle crashes were the leading cause of death for children and teenagers.
- At any given moment, 812,000 vehicles were being driven by someone using a handheld cell phone in the U.S.
- Averages of four children ages 14 and under were killed every day in auto accidents. Nearly 500 were injured daily.
- About 31 percent of fatalities were caused by speeding (10,591).
- Approximately 10% of car accident fatalities were caused by distracted drivers.

- The IIHS says that more than 900 people a year die and nearly 2,000 are injured as a result of vehicles running red lights. About half of those deaths are pedestrians and occupants of other vehicles who are hit by red light runners.
- While fatal car accidents decreased, the number of car accidents resulting in injuries increased 1.9%.
- "Every 10 seconds, someone in the United States is treated in an emergency department for crash-related injuries, and nearly 40,000 people die from these injuries each year. This study highlights the magnitude of the problem of crash-related injuries from a cost perspective, and the numbers are staggering," said Dr. Grant Baldwin, director of CDC's Division of Unintentional Injury Prevention, National Center for Injury Prevention and Control.

A WORLDWIDE PROBLEM

The Global status report on road safety, published by the World Health Organization (WHO), reiterates that road traffic injuries are a global health problem. More than 1.2 million people die on the world's roads every year, and between 20 and 50 million suffer non-fatal injuries. Over 90% of the world's fatalities on the roads occur in low-income and middle-income nations, which have only 48% of the world's vehicles. WHO predicts that road traffic injuries will rise to become the fifth leading cause of death by 2030.

According to the Center for Disease Control (CDC), more than 2.5 million Americans went to the emergency room due to traffic injuries, and nearly 200,000 were then hospitalized in 2012. Americans spend more than 1 million days in the hospital each year from traffic injuries, with a totaled $18 billion in lifetime medical costs. More than 75% of costs occur during the first 18 months following the traffic injury. Lifetime disability for occupants injured in 2012 due to traffic injuries cost an estimated $33 billion.

The incidence and prevalence of "whiplash" varies between different parts of the world, with rates as high as 70 per 100,000 inhabitants in Quebec, Canada, 106 per 100,000 in Australia, and 188 to 325 per 100,000 inhabitants in the Netherlands. According to the World Health Organization, traffic injuries constitute approximately 1% of the combined gross national products of the nations of the western world. Consistent international data indicates that up to 50% of people who sustain a traffic injury will not recover, but will continue to report ongoing pain and disability one year after the injury.

In countries with a very low or non-existent prevalence of late whiplash syndrome or chronic pain from auto collisions, accident victims do not routinely hear reports of acute whiplash leading to chronic symptoms or disability. They do not witness such behavior in others, and do not thereby have any expectation of such possibilities. They do not engage in a process that encourages hypervigilance for and attention to symptoms, thus eliminating many factors that promote symptom amplification and catastrophizing. They also do not engage in a process that engenders anxiety, frustration, fear, and resentment. They do not change their activity in response to what they, after all, view as a minor injury. They will not amplify pre-accident symptoms or symptoms or amplify daily life's aches and pains. They will not attribute all these divergent sources of symptoms to chronic damage they believe the accident caused. There is also no cultural information to encourage the chronic pain behavior present in other cultures.

THE TERM "WHIPLASH" AS A DIAGNOSIS

The term "whiplash" was first used in 1928 by the American orthopedist Crowe, who likened the forces to the crack of a whip when flicked at a high speed. The first wave of such injuries, though, did not involve automobiles. Railway spine became a common diagnosis in the 1800s for people who experienced severe neck pain after being in a train accident. But, because there was no visible trauma to the body, many doctors of the time believed the patients were actually suffering from hysteria, hypochondria, or some other mental illness.

Although widely used by healthcare professions, many find the term whiplash objectionable. Whiplash has gained popularity as a term describing an injury, even though there are no clinical or pathological findings to support it. The diagnosis of whiplash today accounts for an estimated 30 percent of all reported injuries in traffic accidents. Some have started using WAD or Whiplash Associated Disorders which is better but still not accurate.

Reasons why the term whiplash is wrong and should be removed from the medicolegal lexicon:
1. There is a wide spectrum of symptoms and injuries associated with traumatic collisions. Whiplash usually relates to the neck, and does not address the vast potential traffic injuries or symptoms.
2. Whiplash does not accurately represent the various mechanisms of injury seen in traumatic collisions. In 1928, it was thought that the head and neck "whip" back and forth. The Society of Automotive Engineers Paper No. 930889 states that, "Our findings indicate that the time-honored description of the cervical "whiplash" response is both

incomplete and inaccurate." As you will see in the chapter on vehicle damage & occupant injury, the mechanism of injury is much more complicated than just "whiplash".

3. Whiplash is not a technical anatomical diagnosis and is generally associated with minor neck pain. Some traumatic collision injuries are serious and have long term consequences.
4. Whiplash is a jaded term and is often referred to as a "junk" diagnosis.

TRAFFIC INJURIES

The term "Traffic Injuries" is a more appropriate term than "whiplash" to describe the vast number or symptoms and the different mechanisms of injury seen during a collision. Below is a list of common symptoms associated with traffic collisions:

Neck Pain	Sleeping Problems	Hip Pain
Headache	Ringing in the Ears	Leg Pain
Shoulder Pain	Concentration /	Ankle Pain
Middle Back Pain	Memory	Foot Pain
Chest Pain	Dizziness	Sciatica
Low Back Pain	Tinnitus	Paresthesia
Contusions	Difficulty Swallowing	Limited Motion
Arm and Hand Pain	Stress / Anxiety	Vertigo/Dizziness
Numbness	Knee Pain	Hypersensitivity
TMJ Pain	Weakness	Exacerbations
Rib Pain	Muscle Pain	Aggravations
Visual Disturbances	Nerve Pain	
Cognitive Deficits	Radiating pain	

Specific anatomical diagnoses should be determined to explain the reported symptoms.

TRAFFIC COLLISIONS

The majority of traffic collisions could be avoided, if only the drivers would drive more sensibly. Therefore, accidents are not really "accidents," but more properly classified as negligence. About 30% of car accident fatalities occur because of a drunken driver. The majority of car collision victims are the drivers, then the passengers of the car, followed by pedestrians, and lastly cyclists. Every 12 minutes, one person dies because of a car accident. Every 14 seconds, a car accident results in an injured victim.

Traffic injuries can cause any number of different injuries to virtually any part of your body, depending on the conditions of the crash and the severity of the impact. But if you take a closer look at the range of insurance claims and personal injury lawsuits related to auto accidents, you'll see that certain injuries crop up more often than others. The most frequently encountered injuries that result from traffic collisions will be covered in much more detail later in this book.

COMMON CAUSES OF TRAFFIC COLLISIONS

As you now know, traffic collisions are a leading cause of accidental injury and death in the United States, injuring millions and claiming the lives of approximately 30,000 people every year. Understanding the causes of these accidents can help us determine what to do to prevent them.

Distracted driving is one of the leading causes of motor vehicle accidents across the United States. Each day in the U.S., approximately 9 people are killed and more than 1,000 injured in crashes that are reported to involve a distracted driver. Relatively few types of negligent and careless behavior fall under this category, from adjusting the radio to texting while driving. To safely operate a car, truck or any type of motor vehicle, a driver must have complete attention on the matter at hand. The driver's hands must be on the wheel, their eyes on the road, and their mind concentrating on driving. If a single form of the driver's attention is pulled from driving, even for a moment, this can result in a serious accident.

There are three main types of distraction:
- Visual — taking your eyes off the road
- Manual — taking your hands of the wheel
- Cognitive — taking your mind off what you're doing

Distracted driving is any non-driving activity a person engages in while operating a motor vehicle. Such activities have the potential to distract the person from the primary task of driving and increase the risk of crashing. Let's take a look at some statistics concerning distracted driving:

- 10 percent of fatal crashes, 15 percent of injury crashes, and 14 percent of all police-reported motor vehicle traffic crashes in 2015 were reported as distraction-affected crashes.
- In 2015, there were 3,477 people killed and an estimated additional 391,000 injured in motor vehicle crashes involving distracted drivers.
- 9 percent of all drivers 15 to 19 years old involved in fatal crashes were reported as distracted at the time of the crashes. This age group has the largest proportion of drivers who were distracted at the time of the fatal crashes.
- In 2015, there were 551 nonoccupants (pedestrians, bicyclists, and others) killed in distraction-affected crashes.

Speeding is another common cause of traffic collision. In 2015, approximately one-third of fatal auto accidents in the U.S. involved a driver who was exceeding the speed limit or was driving too fast for current conditions (according to statistics from the National Highway Traffic Safety Administration, or NHTSA). Speeding affects a driver's ability to properly control a vehicle, and significantly decreases the amount of time a driver will have to respond to an emergency situation or to stop the vehicle.

Another dangerous practice is drunk driving. About one-third of fatal traffic collisions in 2015 involved at least one driver who had a blood alcohol level of .08% or higher, which is above the legal limit to operate a motor vehicle. Driving under the influence of alcohol affects one's ability to safely operate a vehicle, as it can affect reaction time, motor skills, vision, and the ability to make sound decisions. Additional forms of driver negligence that can lead to collisions include disobeying traffic laws, aggressive driving, and following too closely (tailgating).

No matter its cause, an auto collision has the potential to cause serious injuries and change the lives of everyone involved. That is why I believe it is imperative to do what you can to drive safely, and hopefully avoid being involved in a collision in the first place.

MISCONCEPTIONS AND TRENDS
Recovery from injuries
It is a common myth that everyone suffers long-term pain and disability following a collision. The facts are that, although collisions are traumatic, most people fully recover from their tissue injuries. Of course, trauma is not recommended for a healthy spine, let alone a pathological spine. You will read in later chapters of this book that an accurate diagnosis, hopeful patient expectations, early symptom relief, early joint motion and getting back to normal activity are important in the successful treatment of traffic injuries. Differentiating incidental pathologies from new tissue damage pathologies is also important to prevent chronic pain.

Acute pain is much different than chronic pain. Below are a few of the factors that are predictive that a patient may have a higher risk of developing chronic pain or slower recovery following a traffic collision:
• Initial pain levels of greater than 6/10
• Initial neck disability index scores of greater than 29%
• Symptoms of post-traumatic stress

- Pain catastrophizing
- PTSD
- Recovery Expectations
- Depression
- Cold hyperalgesia

Qualified permanent impairments supported by the AMA Guides to the Evaluation of Permanent Impairment, 6th edition are also indicators for possible prolonged dysfunction or pain.

Rewarding providers

Payers that develop systems for better reimbursement to providers that get good outcomes and do not overutilize care would be very fruitful. Currently payers reward more testing, more treatment, more disability and surgeries by paying more for these claims. There are a small number of providers who have a reputation for doing surgeries, injections, treatment, and imaging, just because it is an injury case, and not because the patient needs the service.

Value-based healthcare is a healthcare delivery model in which providers, including hospitals and physicians, are paid based on patient health outcomes. Under a value-based payment agreement, providers are rewarded for helping patients improve their health, reduce costs, and reduce the incidence of chronic pain.

Self-driving vehicles

We are still many years away, but self-driving vehicles will reduce the number of collisions and, as a result, the number of traffic injuries. Of course, there will be a lag time in the technology and number of early adapters, but this is promising technology over the next 10-20 years. Reducing the number and seriousness of collisions will reduce the number of chronic pain patients.

Incidental Pathologies

Incidental findings on MRI and other diagnostic tests are very common. These findings typically have little to no relation to a patient's complaints. **The facts are that patients with musculoskeletal pain and people without musculoskeletal pain often have similar findings on MRI.** Due to the increase in usage and quality of imaging, doctors are detecting more incidental findings. MRI is widely used as the imaging of choice for musculoskeletal disorders, and may reveal either a clinically insignificant incidental abnormality, or a significant lesion which may explain the patient's symptoms. The provider should treat the patient, not just the scan or tests results.

It is well accepted that x-ray and MRI do not aid prediction of who will or will not experience chronic pain. Most of the herniated discs, facet joint osteoarthritis and other signs of degeneration are very normal, just as grey hair, wrinkles, and getting bald are signs of aging on the outside, disc bulges, facet osteoarthritis, etc., are normal signs of aging on the inside. Below is a table showing age-specific prevalence estimates of degenerative spine imaging findings in asymptomatic patients (Brinjikji, et al., 2015, p. 813):

Imaging Finding	Age (yr)						
	20	30	40	50	60	70	80
Disk degeneration	37%	52%	68%	80%	88%	93%	96%
Disk signal loss	17%	33%	54%	73%	86%	94%	97%
Disk height loss	24%	34%	45%	56%	67%	76%	84%
Disk bulge	30%	40%	50%	60%	69%	77%	84%
Disk protrusion	29%	31%	33%	36%	38%	40%	43%
Annular fissure	19%	20%	22%	23%	25%	27%	29%
Facet degeneration	4%	9%	18%	32%	50%	69%	83%
Spondylolisthesis	3%	5%	8%	14%	23%	35%	50%

Lorimer Moseley, a Professor of Clinical Neurosciences and Chair in Physiotherapy at University of South Australia says, **"If you hurt your back and get an MRI, you've reduced your chances of recovery"**. To go even further, imagine if radiologists added the following sentence after reporting degenerative changes: **"Please note these findings are also commonly seen in asymptomatic populations."** This topic will be discussed more in chapter 4.

Preventing Progressing of Acute Pain to Chronic Pain
There is growing evidence to support that, for many patients with chronic pain, targeting the beliefs and behaviors that drive pain and disability is more effective than simply treating the symptom of pain or incidental findings on MRI. It's in all of our best interest to prevent chronic pain and suffering.

The key components to this approach involve the following:
- Fixing or promote healing of tissue damage.
- Addressing negative beliefs and fear regarding pain and any incidental MRI or x-ray findings.
- Catastrophizing, fear, and worry about pain will actually create the very pain that you fear.
- Providing provider and patient education regarding the mechanisms that drive the vicious cycle of pain and disability.

- Promoting active coping strategies for pain relief and instilling confidence and hope for change.
- Facilitating goal-orientated behavioral change regarding stress management, sleep hygiene, physical activity, exercise, and diet.
- Utilizing motivational and reassurance techniques.
- Training mindfulness of body and movement.
- Monitor responses to pain and movement that perceived as a danger.
- Visual feedback with the use of mirrors, video, and written instruction.
- Identify negative movement and pain behaviors and redirect in a positive direction.
- Targeted motion, strengthening and conditioning.

FURTHER READING TO SUPPORT THIS CHAPTER

Whiplash: evidence base for clinical practice, Michele Sterling PhD, Churchill Livingstone, 2011

Motor Vehicle Collision Injuries, Second Ed, Lawrence Nordhoff, Jones & Bartlett Publishers 2005

National Highway Traffic Safety Administration. Traffic safety facts 2012 data. Washington, DC: US Department of Transportation, National Highway Traffic Safety Administration; 2014.

National Highway Traffic Safety Administration. The economic and societal impact of motor vehicle crashes, 2010. Report no. DOT HS 812 013. Washington, DC: National Highway Traffic Safety Administration; 2014.

Centers for Disease Control and Prevention, National Center for Injury Prevention and Control, Division of Unintentional Injury Prevention.

Crooked: Outwitting the Back Pain Industry and Getting on the Road to Recovery by Cathryn Jakobson Ramin

Traffic Safety Facts Research Note. Report No. DOT HS 812 456). Washington, DC: National Highway Traffic Safety Administration.

Global status report on road safety: time for action. Geneva, World Health Organization, 2009

CHAPTER 2
PAIN

The mechanism of acute pain (tissue damage pain) is not the same as the
mechanism of chronic pain (destructive pain).
Pain really is in the mind, but not in the way you think.
"Use it or lose it", applies to the good and the bad.

SUMMARY – Pain is one of the most common symptoms in the general
population, so it's no surprise that it's commonly reported after a traffic
collision. Pain is largely subjective and has many overlapping causes. Traditional
treatment and management of chronic conditions, including chronic pain, has
been relatively unsuccessful.

Pain does not depend on what is happening in the tissues. Pain depends on
what the brain *thinks* is happening in the tissues.

Pain is defined by the International Association for the Study of Pain as "an
unpleasant sensory and emotional experience associated with actual or
potential tissue damage or described in terms of such damage". Chronic pain is
pain that continues when it should not. The following points are important to
understand about pain:
1. The reporting of pain may or may not involve tissue damage.
2. There is not always a proportional relationship between tissue damage and
pain perception.
3. The relationship between pain and the state of the tissue damage becomes
less predictable the longer pain persists.
4. Our nervous system is plastic (constantly changing).
5. Pain is modulated by many factors from across somatic, psychological and
social realms.
6. Pain should be classified by physiology; acute tissue damage pain (eudynia),
chronic destructive pain (maldynia) or mixed pain.
7. Chronic pain can influence other body systems.
8. To reduce acute pain, we need to reduce the perception of danger and
increase perception of safety in the brain.
9. There is growing evidence to support that, for many patients with chronic
pain, targeting the beliefs and behaviors that drive pain and disability is more
effective than simply treating the symptoms of pain.
10. Preventing acute pain from progressing to chronic pain is essential.

"Pain perception" is the state of being or process of becoming aware of a danger through the senses. The "pain experience" is a mental processing of the pain perception as combinations of thought, perception, memory, emotion, motivation, and imagination. This includes conscious and unconscious brain processes. Catastrophizing, fear, & worry about pain will actually create the very pain that you fear.

Risk of progression to chronic pain:
The majority of patients involved in traffic collisions will recover, but many will have continued symptoms. Important predictors of chronic pain following traffic collisions relate to psychosocial factors and aspects of health, rather than to various attributes of the collision itself. Knowing these factors, and those relating to initial injury severity, it's possible to identify a subgroup of patients presenting with the highest risk of progressing to chronic symptoms. Initial tissue damage, health factors, and psychosocial factors all have an influence on the potential for chronicity. The number and severity of these factors need to be considered in analysis.

Tissue Damage + Health Factors + Psychosocial Factors
Tissue Damage: Injury to skin, muscle, ligament, joint, disc, nerve, bone, brain, cartilage, vascular, eye, ear, or any documentable permanent impairment. The severity of initial damage and any permanent impairment are important to determine.
Health Factors: Any disorder that would increase risk of tissue damage or complicate healing. Examples include fragility, vascular disease, older age, cold hyperalgesia, diabetes, medications, alcoholism, neurological disease, smoking, genetics, nutrition, stenosis, degeneration, RA, lupus, and other conditions.
Psychosocial Factors: Emotions, stress, expectation, anxiety, fear, depression, mental illness, social heredity, job dissatisfaction, catastrophizing, anger, somatization, malingering, secondary gain, conflict, social support, social status, poor treatment selection, fear avoidance, and social integration.

Surprisingly, the bulk of evidence suggests that crash-related factors (e.g. impact direction, awareness of collision, head position) are NOT associated with the prognosis or development of chronic pain.

Neuroplasticity and pain:
Your pain warning system is not just a system for the conduction of pain impulses from the periphery to the brain. Scientists now know that changes can take place in the receptors, nerves, spinal cord, and in the higher brain centers following injury, inflammation, continued use of the pain system, disuse of

inhibiting factors, and learned behaviors. These changes can increase the likelihood that pain is perceived and may contribute to the development of "chronic pain".

The brain and nerve cells that produce pain get better and better at producing pain. They become more and more sensitive and efficient. In other words, neuroplastic changes in structure and function are not only a consequence of chronic pain but are involved in the preservation of pain. Therefore, "chronic pain" can in some cases be considered a separate disease, independent of the pathology that initially set off the pain warning system (alarm system).

Phantom pain is pain that feels like it's coming from a body part that's no longer there. Doctors once believed this post-amputation phenomenon was a psychological problem, but experts now recognize that these real sensations originate in the spinal cord and brain. Chronic pain is not all about the body, and it's not all about the brain and nervous system. It's everything together.

There is good evidence that chronic pain is associated with changes in brain function. It is possible that these brain changes compound chronic pain, and future agents may be able to prevent such complications. German J Psychiatry 2003; 6: 8-15.

The nociceptive (pain) system is not just a system for the conduction of pain impulses from the periphery to the brain. We now know that plastic changes can take place in the periphery, the spinal cord, and also in higher brain centers, following injury or inflammation. These changes may increase the magnitude of the perceived pain, and may contribute to the development of chronic pain syndromes. Swiss Med Wkly 2002;132:273– 278

Emotions change how we perceive pain. Meagher MW, Arnau RC, & Rhudy JL (2001). Pain and emotion: effects of affective picture modulation. Psychosom Med, 63 (1), 79-90

THE PAIN EPIDEMIC

We are truly blessed to live in one of the greatest times in all of human history. Today's modern world allows us all the benefits of heat, air conditioning, internet, refrigeration, transportation, sanitation, security, shelter, science, education, medicine, and much more. Yet, despite these advancements, we have not been able to defeat chronic pain. In fact, chronic pain is now considered to be an epidemic. The Institute of Medicine estimates that 100 million Americans suffer from pain. Pain isn't just an American problem; over

1.5 billion people worldwide suffer from pain. In fact, more people suffer from pain than diabetes, heart disease, stroke, and cancer combined!

Condition	Number of Sufferers:
Pain	100 million people (Institute of Medicine)
Diabetes	20.8 million, diagnosed & estimated undiagnosed (American Diabetes Association)
Coronary Heart Disease and Stroke	18.7 million people (American Heart Association)
Cancer	1.4 million people (American Cancer Society)

Worldwide, pain is a leading cause of disability and a major contributor to health care costs. In the United States, pain is also a significant public health problem that costs society at least $560-$635 billion annually, or equal to $2,000 for everyone living in the US. Lost productivity due to pain costs the US $299-$325 billion, based on factors including days of work missed, hours of work lost, and lower wages. Pain is cited as the most common reason that Americans visit a doctor.

Our past and present paradigms concerning the treatment and management of pain, specifically chronic pain, have been relatively ineffective. It's no surprise then that occupants who have pain after an accident or injury do not get better. This is why a new paradigm is needed. Unfortunately, conventional medicine often has little to offer most pain chronic patients. Even for something as universal as back pain, invasive treatment such as surgery usually is an unsatisfactory first line of care, seconded by prescriptions for opioid painkillers. Approximately 43,000 Americans died in 2016 and 72,000 in 2017 from opioid overdose.

Most chronic pain patients also have other health issues, such as diabetes, obesity, cardiovascular disease, respiratory disease, addictions, asthma, mental health issues, chronic fatigue, arthritis, depression, and many other systemic diseases. Nearly two-thirds of people with chronic pain report problems sleeping, which often makes the pain worse – resulting in a frustrating cycle of pain and sleeplessness. More than half of chronic pain sufferers feel they have little or no control over their pain. Therefore, we must focus on the whole-body health, not just pain relief.

Treating a chronic pain patient can be comparable to fixing a car with four flat tires. You cannot just fix one tire and expect a good result. You must work on all four. In other words, you have to be healthy before you can become healthy.

Although we feel that our views and interventions in modern healthcare are extremely precise and scientific, in many cases that I have reviewed, they are not. The effectiveness of pain treatments depends greatly on the patient, provider, diagnosis, patient selection, patient expectations, healing factors, and the strength of the provider-patient relationship. To reduce pain, we need to reduce the perception of danger and increase credible evidence of safety.

DEFINITION OF PAIN

To get a better understanding of pain, let's start with its definition. The International Association Study of Pain and the AMA Guides have accepted the definition of pain as "an unpleasant sensory and emotional experience associated with actual or potential tissue damage or described in terms of such damage." Pain is a noticeable symptom in many acute injuries and ailments, but often resolves as the disorder resolves. Since acute tissue damage is usually short lived, it is not considered a significant long-term problem.

Chronic pain is defined as pain that persists beyond the expected healing time of the medical disorder thought to have initiated the pain. As a general rule, chronic pain will be the pain that persists beyond 3 months, as most common conditions affecting the musculoskeletal system will markedly heal in this time frame.

Chronic pain is a major health problem, with between 20% and 50% of the population reporting continuous pain for at least 3 of the last 6 months. Chronic pain has been linked with significant disability. Although pain has been traditionally regarded as a symptom that serves a warning signal of an underlying disease process, there is accumulating evidence that persistent pain should be considered a disease entity in its own right. Indeed, permanent changes in the responsiveness of both the peripheral and central nervous systems can persist, even after all tissue healing has ensued; thus, persistent pain can become a self-perpetuating condition.

NOCICEPTIVE PAIN	NEUROPATHIC PAIN	NEUROPLASTIC PAIN
Pain related to *damage* of somatic or visceral tissue, due to trauma or inflammation	Pain related to *damage* of peripheral or central nerves	Pain *without* identifiable nerve or tissue damage.
NOCICEPTIVE PAIN	**NEUROPATHIC PAIN**	**NEUROPLASTIC PAIN**
Examples; Injury, cut or tissue damage	Examples; Painful diabetic peripheral neuropathy, postherpetic neuralgia	Example; Fibromyalgia

Research over the past decade clearly shows that severe or chronic pain leads to abnormal changes in the brain and spinal cord. Central neurologic mechanisms may prolong the experience of pain, even after the inciting factor resolves (tissue damage heals). Researchers and clinicians give a variety of names to this phenomenon—neuropathic pain, neuroinflammatory pain, central sensitization, centrally enhanced pain, centrally mediated pain, embedded pain memory, sympathetic-mediated pain, neuroplastic pain, and brain reorganization. We will refer to it either as chronic pain or maldynia or neuropathic pain.

EUDYNIA (GOOD PAIN) AND MALDYNIA (BAD PAIN)

We usually think of pain in terms of acute injury or inflammation. This type of pain is referred to as eudynia or good pain. This "good" pain can serve a useful purpose, because when we are hurt we also protect ourselves to allow healing and to prevent further damage. This type of pain warns us of tissue damage.

Maldynia or neuropathic pain, on the other hand, has no benefit and is classified as "bad" or chronic pain. It occurs because of abnormal function of the nervous system. The mechanisms of maldynia (bad pain) are substantially different to those of eudynia (good pain). Neuroplastic pain is a form of maldynia (chronic pain). Pain is caused by or increased because of changes within the nervous system. These structural (wiring) and functional (software) changes can occur at every level of the nervous system, including the brain. **It is important to recognize that eudynia (good pain) and maldynia (bad pain) can and often do occur at the same time.**

Nociceptive, acute pain, tissue damage pain or good pain:

Pain that arises from actual or threatened damage to non-neural tissue and is due to the activation of nociceptors. This pain is helpful because it warns the body of tissue damage. This is like an alarm system. Eudynia describes pain occurring with a normally-functioning somatosensory nervous system, rather than the abnormal function seen in neuropathic pain.

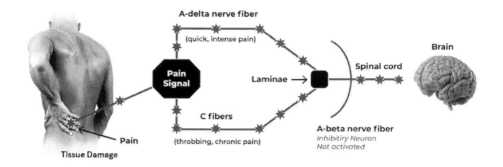

Chronic neuropathic pain or Maldynia (Bad or destructive pain):

Neuropathic pain or maldynia is a complex type of pain initiated or caused by a primary lesion or dysfunction in the nervous system. It is defined as pain arising as a direct consequence of a lesion or pathology affecting the somatosensory system at either the peripheral or central level. Causes of maldynia can be attributed to trauma, surgery, genetics, disease, and processes not yet discovered or understood.

Maldynia is a multidimensional process and a chronic disease, not only affecting sensory and emotional processing, but also producing an alteration of the nervous system. Neural damage to either the peripheral or central nervous system provokes maladaptive responses in pain pathways that generate and magnify pain. It doesn't mean that pain isn't real, or that tissues can't genuinely be in trouble. What it means is that all pain, always, no matter what, is a seriously unreliable interpretation of information coming to your brain from your body.

Neuropathic pain can be triggered by lesions to the somatosensory nervous system that alter its structure and function so that pain occurs spontaneously, and responses to noxious and innocuous stimuli are pathologically amplified. The pain is an expression of maladaptive plasticity within the nociceptive system, a series of changes that constitute a neural disease state. This is also referred to as neuroplastic pain.

Multiple alterations distributed widely across the nervous system contribute to complex pain syndromes. These alterations can occur at any level of the nervous system. Although neural lesions are necessary, they are not sufficient to generate neuropathic pain; genetic alterations, gender, age, and many other factors all influence the risk of developing persistent pain. Treatment needs to move from merely suppressing symptoms to a disease-altering strategy aimed at both preventing or reversing plastic changes and reducing pathology. Below are some common chronic pain conditions:

Central Causes of Neuropathic Pain	Peripheral Causes of Neuropathic Pain
Compression myelopathy due to spinal stenosis	Diabetic neuropathy
HIV myelopathy	Demyelinating polyradiculoneuropathy
Multiple sclerosis pain	Alcoholic polyneuropathy
Pain of Parkinson disease	Complex regional pain syndrome (CRPS)
Myelopathy after ischemia	Entrapment neuropathies
Pain after stroke	HIV sensory neuropathy
Syringomyelia	Idiopathic sensorial neuropathy
Neuroplastic pain	Neuropathy due to nutritional deficiency
	Phantom limb pain
	Post-herpetic neuralgia
	Plexopathy
	Radiculopathy (cervical, thoracic, lumbosacral)
	Neuroplastic pain
	Trigeminal neuralgia
	Post-traumatic neuralgia
	Peripheral nerve injury

Phantom pain
Phantom pain is pain that feels like it's coming from a body part that's no longer there. The sensations of pain originate in the spinal cord and brain. This neurophysiological process can also occur without loss of a body part. In some situations, the brain predicts pain before any tissue damage occurs. We will discuss this in more detail later.

PAIN PERCEPTION
Perception is the brain's best guess about what is happening in the outside world. While the first part of pain perception involves the detecting of potential danger, the second part of pain perception involves the brain evaluating the potential for harm. It is in this second stage that we can calm the warning alarm. The perception of pain is clearly a complex process. It usually acts to tells us when we are potentially damaging our bodies (acute), but sometimes it serves no purpose (chronic).

Individual differences in pain perception has long remained a perplexing and challenging clinical problem. Tissue damage or acute pain has distinct biological and psychological components. The **biology of pain** is the signal transmitted through the central nervous system that "something is wrong." The **psychology of pain** is the interpretation of pain that drives our emotional reactions, thoughts, and behaviors. Suffering results from the emotional responses and perception to pain (stimulus).

First proposed in 1965 by Ronald Melzack and Patrick Wall, the "gate control theory" offers a physiological explanation for the previously observed effect of psychology on pain perception. Although there are some important observations that the gate control theory cannot explain adequately, it remains the theory of pain that most accurately accounts for the physical and psychological aspects of pain perception. The gate control theory provides a neural basis which reconciled the specificity and pattern theories and ultimately revolutionized pain research. Despite flaws in its presentation of neural architecture, the theory of gate control is currently the only theory that most accurately accounts for the physical and psychological aspects of pain.

Following an injury, pain signals are transmitted to the spinal cord and then up to the brain. There is a "gate" in your spinal cord that determines whether or not the signals will be passed to the brain. The "gate control theory" of pain asserts that non-painful input closes the "gates" to painful input, which prevents pain sensation from traveling to the central nervous system. Therefore, stimulation by non-noxious input is able to suppress pain.

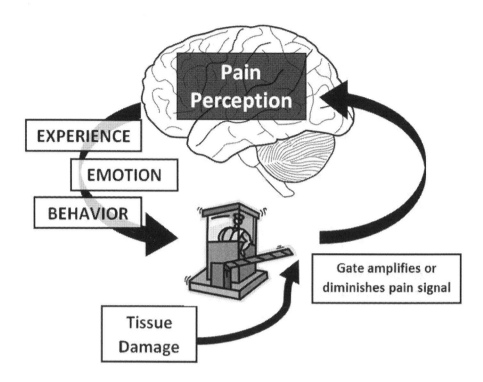

These gates can sometimes be much more open than at other times (causing more pain). If the gates are more open, then a lot of pain messages pass through to the brain, and you are likely to experience a high level of pain. If the gates are more closed, then fewer messages get through, and you are likely to experience less pain.

Examples of therapies that close the gate (stop pain) are: topical analgesics, joint manipulation, massage, acupuncture, electrical stimulation, traction, compression, thermal stimulation (ice / heat), contrast bath, TENS, exercise, and motion. Feeling generally happy and optimistic has been found to help to close the gates to pain. Also, feeling relaxed in yourself seems to be a particularly useful way of closing the gates. Concentrating on something other than pain (e.g. working, gardening, reading) can distract you from any pain, helping to close the gates.

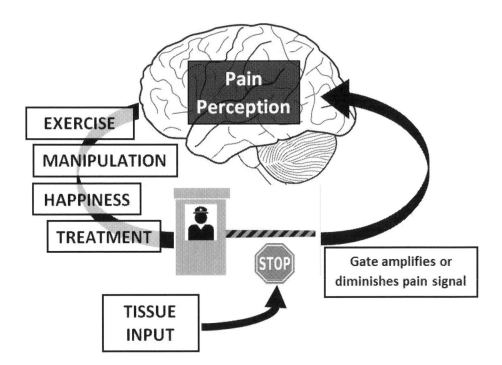

There are three main ways in which the gates to pain can be made more open, so that the pain feels worse: emotional states, focusing on the pain, and lack of activity. Emotional states can lead to the gates to pain being more open. These include being anxious, worried, angry, and depressed. Having a lot of tension in the body is a common way of opening the pain gates. Mentally focusing on the pain is one of the most powerful ways of opening the gates and increasing your pain. Other factors that have been shown to open the pain gates are lack of movement or activity, stiff joints, boredom, and lack of fitness.

A recent study at Northwestern University's Feinberg School of Medicine found that chronic pain also changes the way information is processed in the brain. In the healthy brains, all regions existed in a state of equilibrium – when one region was active, the others quieted down. But in those with chronic pain, a front region of the cortex mostly associated with emotion "never stops". The region was stuck on full throttle, wearing out neurons and altering their connections to each other.

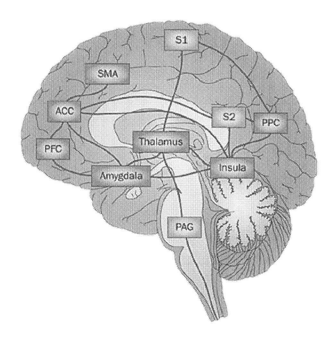

The study also revealed two interesting factors that may contribute to chronic pain. First, the nucleus accumbens is an important center for teaching the rest of the brain how to evaluate and react to the outside world. What this means is that this area of the brain may actually use the pain signal to teach the rest of the brain to develop chronic pain. Second, the participants in the research study lost gray matter density in their brains, which is likely linked to fewer synaptic connections, which are essential for communication between neurons.

It helps to see the brain and the nervous system as the central alarm center, continuously protecting (consciously and subconsciously) the body from its environment, body, and past experiences. Chronic pain can be viewed as an alarm system not functioning properly. To turn off the alarm (reduce pain), we need to reduce the perception of danger and increase the reality of safety.

In some cases, injury by itself is not enough to explain the ongoing pain. It has to do with the injury combined with the state of the brain and psychological factors. Some areas of the brain are more excited in certain individuals to begin with, or there may be genetic and environmental influences that predispose these brain regions to interact at an excitable level. There are many different factors that influence the experience of pain, which is different for everyone. These include: age, gender, culture, ethnicity, spiritual beliefs, socio-economic status, emotional response, support systems, life before pain onset, learned response from family, societal systems, and medical care providers.

NEUROPLASTICITY

Pain is much more than just a sensation caused by a specific stimulus (tissue damage). Pain is a complex neurological function with physical, emotional, and cognitive components. Our nervous system controls or has a part in every function of our body. The nervous system also has the amazing ability to adapt and change. This is called neuroplasticity. Neuroplasticity updates the operating functions of the nervous system, both structurally and functionally.

Neuroplasticity is a mechanism whereby the physical anatomy and physiological parts of the nervous system adapts to conditions. This is the hardware and software for our nervous system (our computer). It is programmable, and when neuroplastic changes occur, they cause both physical changes and physiological changes in the neurological patterns of operation. In many ways, our pain system is similar to a home alarm system.

Neuroplasticity is generally very good for us; we learn a trade or career, we develop balance, we learn math, we learn to play baseball or the piano, and thousands of other functions we do every day that we do not even think about. There is also a bad side of neuroplasticity that deals with bad habits, addictions, certain diseases, and in many cases, pain.

The good thing is that, "Between stimulus and response there is a pause. In that pause is our power to choose our response. In our response lie our growth and our freedom." This choice takes place in a region of the brain called the prefrontal cortex. A good illustration of this control is the expression, "Your mind is a wonderful servant, but a horrible master".

VERY BASIC NEUROLOGY

For our discussion, the nervous system will be anatomically divided into three sections; the central nervous system (CNS), peripheral nervous system (PNS), and a branch of the PNS called the enteric nervous system (ENS). The central nervous system is made up of the brain and spinal cord. The peripheral nervous system basically consists of everything else but is further divided into the somatic and the autonomic nervous systems. The enteric nervous system is technically part of the autonomic nervous system of the PNS, but due to its clinical significance we will be discussing it more in-depth.

CENTRAL NERVOUS SYSTEM (BRAIN AND SPINAL CORD)

The brain and spinal cord are what we typically think of as the nervous system. They both are encapsulated and protected by bone. The brain is considered the control center of the body. The spinal cord is the main line or connection from the brain to the rest of the body. Think of your brain as a mega supercomputer, and the spinal cord as a fiber optic cable bundle. The spinal cord is our life line. Without it, the brain loses much of its communication with the rest of the body. There are also reflexes that occur in our spinal cord that are essential for our body to function.

Your brain is approximately three pounds of soft gray matter divided down the middle into two halves. Your brain is approximately 80 percent water. The brain accounts for about 2 percent of the body's weight, yet it receives approximately 20% of total body oxygen consumption, 15% of the cardiac output, and 25% of total body glucose utilization. The central nervous system contains more than 100 billion neurons and processes millions of bits of information every second. The brain is broken up into parts for study and diagnostic purposes, but it functions as one amazing structure.

The brain is responsible functions such as; perception, attention, memory, emotion, learning, coordination of sensory systems, respiration, fine motor skills, walking, vision, hearing, smell, blood pressure, fluid balance, reading, body temperature, respiration, heart rate, and much more. The brain does millions of functions at any given time just to keep us alive. The brain is truly amazing, but one area of the brain is particularly important for pain relief. This area is called the frontal lobe.

The frontal lobe (pre-frontal cortex) is the general area of brain that has been found to play a role in the "executive functions" of the entire nervous system. The centers for judgment, speech, emotions, complex thought, language, memory, motor function, socialization, planning, personality, sensory functions, and behavior are all located in the frontal lobe. This area has the ability to override and suppress or stimulate other areas of the nervous and endocrine systems. There is also a rich neuronal input from the alert centers of the brain-stem, and limbic regions. So, this is the central command center for the whole body.

PERIPHERAL NERVOUS SYSTEM (NERVES OR WIRES)
The peripheral nervous system (PNS) for the most part consists of everything except the brain and spinal cord. The PNS transmits messages to and from the central nervous system. It is further divided into the somatic and the autonomic nervous systems. The somatic nervous system is responsible for carrying sensory information from the body to the brain and coordinating movement. It is the system that regulates activities that are under conscious control by the

brain – in other words, we have some control over it. Theses nerves relay orders from the brain to the body or transmit sensory information to the brain from the body.

The autonomic nervous system regulates activities unconsciously, or without us knowing about it. The autonomic nervous system is split into 3 divisions: the sympathetic division, parasympathetic division, and enteric division. The sympathetic nervous system responds to danger or stress, and is responsible for increased heart rate. The parasympathetic nervous system, on the other hand, is evident when a person is resting and feels relaxed and is responsible for such things as the constriction of the pupil, the slowing of the heart, the dilation of the blood vessels, and the stimulation of the digestive and genitourinary systems.

ENTERIC NERVOUS SYSTEM

The gut truly has a mind of its own and it's called the enteric nervous system (ENS). Just like the brain in the head this system sends and receives impulses, records experiences and respond to emotions. Its nerve cells are bathed and influenced by the same neurotransmitters as the rest of the nervous system. The role of the enteric nervous system is to manage every aspect of digestion, from the esophagus to the stomach, small intestine and colon.

The enteric nervous system is often referred to as "the second brain", is a part of the peripheral nervous system and a division of the autonomic nervous system which controls the gastrointestinal tract. This system of afferent and efferent connections with the central nervous system (CNS) is not only complex and integrated, but is also capable of autonomous function, controlling the digestive system in the context of the physiological state locally, and the body as a whole.

The gut's brain, or simply the "ENS," is located in the sheaths of tissue lining the esophagus, stomach, small intestine, and colon. Although the ENS communicates with the brain, its complex circuitry enables it to act independently, learn, remember and is responsible for "gut feelings".

The ENS also plays a major role in human happiness and misery. Many gastrointestinal disorders like colitis and irritable bowel syndrome originate from problems within the enteric nervous system. Pay attention to your gut-brain connection – it may contribute to your anxiety and digestion problems. The gut contains 100 million neurons (more than the spinal cord). Major neurotransmitters like serotonin, dopamine, glutamate, norepinephrine, and nitric oxide are in the gut. Also, two dozen small brain proteins called neuropeptides are there, along with the major cells of the immune system.

A higher-than-normal percentage of people with IBS (irritable bowel syndrome) and intestinal problems develop chronic pain, depression or anxiety. This is very important because a large percent of the population has functional bowel problems. The brain, gut and diet are intricately connected, and communicate in a tri-directional manner. In other words, it's a 3-way intersection, meaning that diet, stress and pain can cause problems with the gut and problems with the gut can cause stress and pain.

FUNCTIONAL OVERVIEW (SOFTWARE)

It is important to point out that, although we divide the body and the nervous system into parts to better understand anatomy, physiology, and disease, in reality the nervous system and body function as one complete system, with your nervous system having constant communication and feedback with virtually every aspect of your body. Your brain also catalogs or saves information and memories to make future decisions.

The more you learn about the nervous system, the more amazed and impressed you will be. The brain is the central command center for most of your bodily processes. Everything that you see, feel, hear, smell, taste, touch, or think is brought to the attention of the brain. This includes pain. Your brain tells you about the different aspects of pain including location, severity, frequency, and different qualities of pain. Since the brain controls our perception of pain, you are able to use your brain to influence pain. Specific areas of the nervous system that deal with pain have been studied and identified. These areas include the pain receptors, nerves that carry pain, reflexes in the spinal cord, and areas of the brain that deal with pain.

In our nervous system, different types of receptors provide us with information such as touch, smell, vision, balance, taste, pressure, pain, and many other "feelings". These receptors send information using peripheral nerves (wires) to the spinal cord (the main wire). Once in the spinal cord, reflexes occur and the information continues up the spinal cord to the brain. The brain receives the information and relays it to different areas within the brain. All this occurs in a fraction of a second, without us even thinking about it. The message is delivered, interpreted, and then acted on.

The nervous system can also "predict" or anticipate different sensations, even pain. For instance, you think a cup has orange juice in it and pick the cup up to drink it. Instead of orange juice, the cup has milk in it. Your brain predicts the taste of orange juice and, for a split second, the milk tastes like orange juice. Another example is when you smell some food that makes your mouth "water" (secrete saliva), preparing you to eat. Or, if you get an injection and see the needle coming, you may feel the "prick" before the needle even touches your skin.

Another fascinating thing about the brain is that it catalogs all life experiences, whether real or observed. Your brain does not differentiate between watching something on television and an actual experience. Your brain still catalogs it for information purposes to be recalled at a later date. How many times have you heard, "Well, I saw it on TV"? This is why it is important to guard what we think, see, and hear to prevent negative mental programming.

The "hard wired" view of the nervous system is very practical for learning, but is not correct. In reality, the nervous system is very complicated and dynamic. The nervous system is obsessed with stimulation, adaptation, and efficiency. For example, the more you play the piano, kick a soccer ball, shoot a basketball, read braille, ride a bike, drive a car, or do thousands of other things, the more your brain learns. The brain learns new processes so well that an activity can be "trained" to be performed on autopilot. Have you ever driven home without thinking about the roads to take, or typed without looking at the keys? We develop habits and addictions all the time, and we do not even realize it. Some habits are good for us and some are bad for us.

We know that the brain catalogs and organizes your experiences, sensations, emotions, and thoughts. The brain uses this information for responses to future events and, over time, can develop habits or addictions. Your brain may also use the stored information to predict or anticipate future events. The brain does all this automatically and instinctively. The frontal lobe is the area of the brain that gives you the conscious ability to override the body's unconscious responses, reflexes, habits, or addictions. You have the power to be in control, but you must consciously work to make changes.

Our nervous system is one of the most amazing and complicated structures in the universe. The brain and nervous system remain a dynamic structure that alters from year-to-year, day-to-day, even moment-to-moment, over our lifespan. Your brain catalogs and organizes all of your experiences, sensations, emotions, and thoughts. It uses this information and data to make future decisions. The frontal lobe (pre-frontal cortex) is the general area of brain that has been found to play a role in the "executive functions" of the entire nervous system.

While DNA helps to determine what kind of brain you start with, your life experiences (and epigenetics) determine how your brain will develop and work over your lifetime. Your nervous system never stops learning and adapting, but the early years are the most important. This is when we lay the framework for our "neural network". Amazingly, we are born with an excess of brain cells. These excess cells and neural connections in the brain die off when they are not stimulated. The saying, "use it or lose it" is a neurological fact. Each person is wired differently, because each person has a different combination of life's experiences.

Neuroplasticity refers to the changes that occur in the organization of your nervous system as a result of your experiences, thoughts, and actions. Each time we have a neurological event, the brain creates either a new synaptic connection (new memory) or reuses an old synaptic connection (old memory). If you do not use these connections, the unused connections will simply die off; conversely, the more you use a connection, the more efficient the process gets. *Repetition is the mother of all learning.*

USE IT OR LOSE IT!

The brain is made up of tiny nerve cells called neurons. These neurons have tiny, branch-like structures that reach out and connect with other neurons. Each place where a neuron connects with another neuron is called a synapse, or synaptic connection. The pattern and way our neurons connect to each other forms our "neural network". These connections form our ideas, thoughts, and memories. Every single connection has an influence on our future thoughts and actions. Billions of neurons communicate across these synapses, allowing every thought, sensation, and event to be trace (new memory) or retrace (old memory) neural pathways. There may be only a few hundred or as many as 200,000 such synaptic connections to each neuron.

The more you use a neurological connection, the stronger it gets. If you stop using the connection, the neurons are pruned away. Use it or lose it!

The more neural connections and synapses (repetition) you have for a particular sensation or function, the stronger the synapse is neurologically. Your brain also connects smells, sounds, feelings, emotions, and other sensations which also make the neural connections stronger. The brain is considered "neuroplastic," or changing, because it responds to life experiences and then alters its structure and function. Our brain is constantly learning, altering, and adapting, but the

33

more you use and re-trace parts of your "neural network", the more "hard wired" or automatic the function appears to be. "Use it or lose it," "practice makes perfect," and "repetition is the mother of all learning," are not just expressions. They are neurological facts.

Knowledge allows you to become aware of the brain's power to change and become the observer. Neuroplasticity makes it easier to do some things "automatically," but it is also why habits or addictions are difficult to break. How does neuroplasticity relate to pain? How can you use neuroplasticity to your advantage?

If we have a new experience, the neurons make new synaptic connections or trace new pathways. If we have an experience that has already been traced, then the neurons use already established pathway or retrace the pathway. The more a synaptic connection is used, the easier it is retraced. If you practice something over and over, you are re-wiring and strengthening your "neural network." You can also break synaptic connections by not using the neuro pathway. Neural pruning is the term that is used to describe neurons dying off when not being used. In other words – use it or lose it.

The complexity of our "neural network" is almost beyond comprehension. Over a lifetime, each person will have different experiences, thoughts, ideas, values, and education. It is this "neural network" that shapes our present and future thoughts, opinions, and actions. The more synaptic connections we have relating to experiences of pain, learned or observed, the more we feel or associate with pain.

GENETICS AND EPIGENETICS

Genetics play a role in everything from hair color to complicated disease processes. It's widely accepted that genetic factors are important contributors to individual differences in pain sensitivity, anatomical variations, anxiety, and risk for developing painful conditions.

Epigenetics, in a simplified definition, is the study of biological mechanisms that will switch genes on and off. Certain circumstances in life can cause genes to be silenced or expressed over time. In other words, they can be turned off (becoming dormant) or turned on (becoming active). The good news is that this means that each individual has more control over their genetic expression than previously thought.

Growing interest in epigenetics and the genetics of pain will accelerate advances in the field. We will understand more how interactions between multiple genes and epigenetics shape the human experience of pain and progression from acute to chronic pain. The field of genetics and the role in pain is still in its early stages.

SOCIAL INHERITANCE

The nature versus nurture debate is one of the oldest philosophical issues within psychology. Nature refers to all of the genetic factors that influence who we are, including pain and health. Nurture refers to all the social and environmental variables that impact who we are, including our early childhood experiences, how we were raised, our social relationships, and our surrounding culture. Nurture can also be referred to as our social inheritance, because the strongest traits are learned early in life. This is a very important and often overlooked aspect of our neuroplastic makeup.

Through studies with identical twins separated at birth, scientists have discovered that approximately 40% of our health and happiness is determined by our social hereditary. Thus, the key to health and happiness lies not in changing our genetic makeup and not in changing our life circumstances, but in our daily behavior. It's also important to point out that our behavior has an influence on turning on & off our genes (epigenetics).

THE EXPERIENCE OF PAIN IS COMPLICATED

If "pain" posted its relationship status with us on a social media site, it would read, "it's complicated". Pain, injury, and chronic pain are multifaceted, intertwined, and complex. There are many aspects of pain that we don't yet know that we don't know. However, we do know that poor recovery after traffic injury has been constantly reported to be related with high initial pain intensity, pain-related disability, posttraumatic stress, pain catastrophizing, fear avoidance, fear of motion, poor expectations of recovery, and passive coping.

Severe tissue damage, health factors, and psychosocial factors also all have an influence on the potential for chronicity. Transition of acute to chronic pain may be minimized by early recognition of risk factors for chronicity. To reduce pain in the nervous system, we need to reduce the perception of danger and increase perception of safety. Below is my pain experience scale indicating some factors and the cumulative effect factors associated with chronic pain.

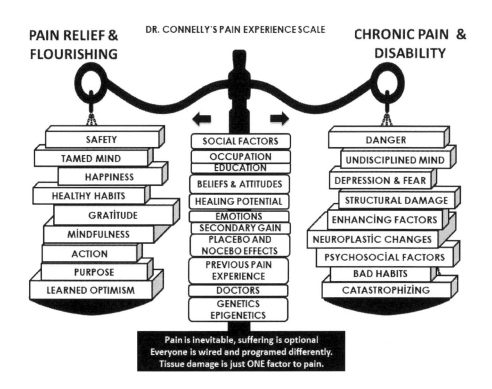

Dr. Connelly's Pain Experience Scale

PAIN RELIEF & FLOURISHING

| SAFETY |
| TAMED MIND |
| HAPPINESS |
| HEALTHY HABITS |
| GRATITUDE |
| MINDFULNESS |
| ACTION |
| PURPOSE |
| LEARNED OPTIMISM |

| SOCIAL FACTORS |
| OCCUPATION EDUCATION |
| BELIEFS & ATTITUDES |
| HEALING POTENTIAL |
| EMOTIONS |
| SECONDARY GAIN |
| PLACEBO AND NOCEBO EFFECTS |
| PREVIOUS PAIN EXPERIENCE |
| DOCTORS |
| GENETICS EPIGENETICS |

CHRONIC PAIN & DISABILITY

| DANGER |
| UNDISCIPLINED MIND |
| DEPRESSION & FEAR |
| STRUCTURAL DAMAGE |
| ENHANCING FACTORS |
| NEUROPLASTIC CHANGES |
| PSYCHOSOCIAL FACTORS |
| BAD HABITS |
| CATASTROPHIZING |

Pain is inevitable, suffering is optional
Everyone is wired and programed differently.
Tissue damage is just ONE factor to pain.

DEFINITIONS TO SUPPORT THIS CHAPTER

Eudynia - "the good"; acute nociceptive pain; a symptom; useful; warning pain; tissue damage pain. This pain is helpful because it warns the body of tissue damage. Commonly referred to as nociceptive or acute pain.

Nociceptive (Eudynia) pain - Pain that arises from actual or threatened damage to non-neural tissue and is due to the activation of nociceptors. The term is used to describe pain occurring with a normally functioning somatosensory nervous system to contrast with the abnormal function seen in neuropathic or acute pain.

Maldynia - "the bad"; destructive; sensitization of the nervous system; usually chronic pain, no benefits to the person; pain becomes the disease process itself (neuropathic pain).

Neuropathic pain (Maldynia) - Pain caused by a lesion or disease of the somatosensory nervous system at either the peripheral or central level. Continual maldynia; LAPS, CRPS, phantom pain, myofascial pain, IBS, fibromyalgia, chronic headaches, chronic mood changes.

Neuroplastic Pain (Maldynia) - Classified as a form of neuropathic pain or maldynia. Refers to pain caused by or pain increased because of changes within the nervous system. These structural and functional changes can occur at every level of the nervous system.

Nociplastic pain (Maldynia) - Pain that arises from altered nociception despite no clear evidence of actual or threatened tissue damage causing the activation of peripheral nociceptors or evidence for disease or lesion of the somatosensory system causing the pain.

Pain Processing - The physiology of pain involves activation and complex interactions of autonomic, peripheral, and central nervous systems, as well as endocrine and immune systems.

Nociceptor - a sensory receptor for painful stimuli.

Noxious stimulus - A stimulus that is damaging or threatens damage to normal tissues.

A-alpha nerve fibers - carry information related to proprioception (muscle sense).

A-beta nerve fibers - carry information related to touch (mechanical stimulation). One phenomenon you may have observed in yourself is that stimulation of touch sensors (A-beta fibers) in the skin by rubbing can disrupt the sensation of pain arising in a nearby structure such as a muscle. This is usually interpreted in terms of the gate control theory.

A-delta nerve fibers - carry information related to pain, pressure and temperature. Sharp acute pain.

C-nerve fibers - carry information related to pain, noxious heat and chemical stimulation. Unmyelinated and have a small diameter, poor pain localization and low conduction velocity. C fiber can respond to a broad range of painful stimuli, including mechanical, thermal or metabolic factors.

Sensitization - Increased responsiveness of nociceptive neurons to their normal input, and/or recruitment of a response to normally subthreshold inputs.

Categories of Pain Fibers		
Type	Size and Description	Pain Response
A-β Fibers	Large skin nerve fibers	Non-nociceptive pain, proprioceptors
A-δ Fibers	Smaller Myelinated skin fibers that play an important role in the localization of noxious stimulation	Mechanoreceptive pain; hyperalgesia; quick, intense, acute pain
C Fibers	Small, unmyelinated fibers; represent 75% of peripheral nerve fibers	Nociceptive: throbbing, burning, chronic pain

Pain Threshold - The least experience of pain which a subject can recognize.

Pain Tolerance Level - The greatest level of pain which a subject is prepared to tolerate.

Analgesia - Absence of pain in response to stimulation which would normally be painful.

Hypoalgesia - Diminished pain in response to a normally painful stimulus.

Allodynia - Pain due to or resulting from a stimulus which does not normally provoke pain.

Hyperalgesia - Extreme sensitivity to pain; greater than normal sensitivity to pain.

Hyperpathia - Clinical symptom/sign of neurological disorder whereby a painful stimulus evokes greater pain than would be expected, i.e. a pin prick feels like a knife.

Referred Pain Patterns - Pain felt in one part of the brain/body due to pathology in a different part of the brain/body, such as a heart attack causing left arm pain. There are no nerves directly from the heart to the left arm. However, nerves from the heart and nerves from the left arm go essentially the same place in the spinal cord. When the message gets up to the brain, the brain may not know where the pain is really coming from.

Neuroplasticity - refers to the ability of the nervous system to alter its structure and function. Neuroplasticity (also deals with brain plasticity, cortical plasticity and cortical re-mapping) refers to changes that occur in the organization of the brain and entire nervous system as a result of experiences. "Plasticity" relates to the learning by adding or removing connections, or cells.

Neural Pruning - Our brain is actively pruning away (getting rid of) neural connections that we don't use.

Brain Plasticity - the ability of the brain to modify its connections or re-wire itself.

Prefrontal Cortex (PFC) - Executive center of the brain. Most anterior or front part of the brain. It plays an important role in cognitive control, in the ability to orchestrate thought, action, and self-control.

Amygdala - A limbic brain area, the amygdala plays a key role in emotional responses and affective states and disorders such as learned fear, anxiety, and depression. The amygdala has also emerged as an important brain center for the emotional-affective dimension of pain and for pain modulation.

"Name it to tame it" - Naming a fear, stress, or emotion activates the prefrontal cortex (executive center) and calms the limbic amygdala (pain, stress, depression, and fear centers).

Psychosomatic pain - a physical disease that is thought to be caused or made worse by mental factors. Placebo and nocebo effects are presumably psychogenic, but they can induce measurable changes in the body and the brain.

Nocebo (I shall harm) - Negative expectations deriving from clinical encounters can produce negative outcomes. For example, an expectation of pain may induce anxiety which, in turn, causes the release of cholecystokinin, which facilitates pain transmission.

Nocebo effect - is the induction of a symptom perceived as negative by sham treatment and/or by the suggestion of negative expectations.

Nocebo response - is a negative symptom induced by the patient's own negative expectations and/or by negative suggestions from clinical staff in the absence of any treatment.

Placebo (I please) - a substance that may produce a beneficial, healthful, pleasant, or desirable effect.

FURTHER READING TO SUPPORT THIS CHAPTER

Neuroplasticity - an important factor in acute and chronic pain. Swiss Med Wkly 2002;132:273– 278

Basbaum, Allan. (2002). Pain physiology: basic science. Canadian Journal of Anesthesia/Journal canadien d'anesthésie. 49. R1-R3. 10.1007/BF03018125.

May, Arne. (2009). New insights into headache: An update on functional and structural imaging findings. Nature reviews. Neurology.

Enck, Paul; Benedetti, Fabrizio; Schedlowski, Manfred (July 2008). "New Insights into the Placebo and Nocebo Responses". Neuron. 59 (2): 195–206.

The Brain and Chronic Pain. German J Psychiatry 2003; 6: 8-15

Whiplash-associated disorder: musculoskeletal pain and related clinical findings. J Man Manip Ther. 2011 Nov; 19(4): 194–200.

Genetic predictors of human chronic pain conditions. Neuroscience 338 (2016) 36–62.

No man is an island: Living in a disadvantaged neighborhood influences chronic pain development after motor vehicle collision. Pain 155 (2014) 2116–2123.

Polymorphisms in the glucocorticoid receptor co-chaperone FKBP5 predict persistent musculoskeletal pain after traumatic stress exposure. Pain. 2013 August ; 154(8): 1419–1426.

Incidence and predictors of neck and widespread pain after motor vehicle collision among US litigants and nonlitigants. PAIN 155, Issue 2, (2014), Pages 309–321.

An Overview of Systematic Reviews on Prognostic Factors in Neck Pain: Results from the International Collaboration on Neck Pain (ICON) Project. The Open Orthopaedics Journal, 2013, 7, (Suppl 4: M9) 494-505.

Genetic predictors of acute and chronic pain. Edwards, R.R. Curr Rheumatol Rep (2006) 8: 411.

Recovery Pathways and Prognosis After Whiplash Injury. J Orthop Sports Phys Ther 2016;46(10):851–861.

Rehabilitation of the Spine: A Practitioner's Manual Second Edition by Craig Liebenson DC

CHAPTER 3
VEHICLE DAMAGE & OCCUPANT INJURY (ACUTE PAIN)

Whether or not a person sustains an injury is a function of multiple factors. Each person has a different tolerance to trauma or potential for tissue damage. The risk factors for acute symptoms are not the same as the risk factors for chronic symptoms.

SUMMARY – "Whether or not a victim sustains an injury is a function of multiple factors: the magnitude of the impact, their posture at the time, their anatomy, and the material strength of the components of their cervical spine." Biomechanics of Musculoskeletal Injury, 2ed, William Whiting PhD, Ronald Zernicke PhD, 2008, page 269

"A common misconception formulated is that the amount of vehicle crash damage due to a collision offers a direct correlation to the degree of occupant injury. The paper explores this concept and explains why it is false reasoning. Explanations with supporting data are set forth to show how minor vehicle damage can relate or even be the major contributing factor to occupant injury. Mathematical equations and models also support these findings." Malcolm C. Robbins (1997) Society of Automobile Engineers "Lack of relationship between vehicle damage and occupant injury." 97-02-01: (#970494): 117-9

Collision Factors + Human Factors = Risk of Acute Injury

The external forces, momentum, angle, velocity, secondary impacts, acceleration, and deceleration for each collision are unique to each occupant. Based on scientific and medical literature, there are two major factors that determine an occupant's risk for acute injury: human risk factors and collision factors, or forces imposed on the occupant during the collision. The risk factors for acute symptoms are not the same as the risk factors for chronic symptoms.

INTRODUCTION

Traffic collisions are a source of pain and injury to many people every year, but the existence of these injuries causally related to the collision is often challenged. Accident reconstructionists and biomechanical analysis definitely provides helpful information, yet the science does not provide an absolute correlation between vehicle damage and occupant injury. Over my 20 years in practice, I have seen patients involved in very serious collisions with no significant injury and others with very little vehicle damage but reports extensive pain. This raises the questions: "If the vehicle did not suffer any damage, how could the occupant become injured?" or, "If the vehicle suffered significant damage, how could the occupant walk away with little to no injury?"

Some patients improve, and some patients develop chronic conditions. Why? First of all, each collision and each occupant are unique. Evaluation must be objective and based on the individual, the unique factors of the collision, and the potential to cause injury to that occupant. The physical and psychological components of a collision are unique to each occupant.

Over the past 70 years, hundreds of research studies have sought to detail the mechanisms involved in auto collisions. These studies have involved use of live subjects, cadaveric studies, computer simulations, electromyography, and mathematical modeling. As a result of these studies, we have a better understanding of collision dynamics and the varied mechanisms of injury. Vehicle crashworthiness, ridged bumper systems, certain body frames, and impacts with greater mass will often have more energy available to impose on the occupant.

The collision and subsequent forces imposed on the occupants are unquestionably one factor for assessment, but there are many other factors to take into consideration. There is no absolute linear or direct correlation between vehicular damage and occupant injury. Traffic collisions are complex events, and during a collision one person may be injured, while another who may even be in the same car may be symptom-free. Using the cost to repair a vehicle or a few pictures of vehicle damage often does not provide the necessary information needed to determine occupant injury.

Traffic collision related injuries are the most frequently litigated type of injury in the United States, primarily due to two facts: Traffic collisions are one of the most common sources of injuries in our society, and many traffic related injuries result from negligence of another individual. Worldwide, traffic collisions lead to death and disability, as well as financial costs to both society and the individuals involved.

Individuals involved in traffic accidents can be held financially liable for the consequences of an accident, including property damage, injuries to passengers and drivers, and fatalities. Because these damages can easily exceed the annual income of the average driver, most US states require drivers to carry liability insurance to cover these potential costs. Claims of injury naturally produce a polar alignment of opinion, with one side favoring the claimant and the other side favoring the defense.

The likelihood of significant injury arising from a low-speed rear impact collision is the subject of scholarly debate, but in the real world, each collision, each occupant, and each risk of injury is unique. There are several basic biomechanical engineering principles that we will discuss in this chapter. When considering injury causation and any subsequent post-traumatic disorders, it is imperative for the physician or any evaluator to remember that there is no "typical" human in a real-world crash environment. There are many human and collision variables that help to determine an occupant's risk of acute injury. We will also discuss some of the factors associated with progression to chronic conditions or poor prognosis.

"POSSIBLE" VS "PROBABLE"

It's difficult to discuss vehicle damage and occupant injury without discussing possible and probable, causation, and apportionment.

A causal relationship between a trauma and an injury is defined as "probable" if the cause and effect relationship is greater than 50% ("more likely than not"). There is a "possible" causal relationship between the alleged cause and an event when the likelihood is a causal relationship is equal to or less than 50%. A reasonable degree of medical probability or certainty, then, simply means that something is more likely to occur than not (probability exceeds 50%). On the other hand, the probability of an event's occurrence equal to or less than 50% is just a possibility.

Just because there was a collision does not mean that all the pain, symptoms, or tissue damage resulted from the impact. Whereas it's possible for injuries to occur from traffic collisions, the facts must demonstrate that the "possible" is in fact "probable." In some cases, there may be more than one cause of the symptoms, and apportionment is needed. Apportionment is simply a distribution of causation among multiple factors that caused or significantly contributed to the injury or disease and resulting impairment.

There are also cases that are anomalies and seem inconsistent with the facts but have no other explanation. For example, a professional baseball player tore his lateral collateral ligament in his right knee, which he sustained while attempting to take off his shoe. "Smith said he was getting ready to shower after pitching in a minor league game on Thursday and was standing on one leg to take off his other shoe when he lost his balance and twisted the knee." It was later found out that he tore ligaments. These types of injuries are rare, but it stresses the importance that each claim of injury should be evaluated individually.

CAUSATION

A superficial determination of causation can be found in the American Medical Association: Guides to the Evaluation of Permanent Impairment, sixth edition, page 25. Causality requires determination that each of the following has occurred to a reasonable degree of medical certainty:

- A causal event took place.
- The patient experiencing the event has the condition.
- The event could cause the condition.
- The event caused or materially contributed to the condition within medical probability.

A more comprehensive look into a causal relationship one must determine if the requirements of temporal relationship, biologic plausibility, literature support, and sufficient injury have been met. There must be a probable relationship between the trauma and the symptoms. The central issue is whether a particular collision (trauma) would cause the claimed tissue damage. To determine this, one must assess the following elements:

1. A temporal relationship between the trauma and injury. **Temporality is one of the strongest evidences of causation in evaluating a patient.** To determine this, one must make judgements that refer to:

      a. the time interval between the trauma and the symptom appearance,

      b. variation of symptoms with time.

2. What is the injury (tissue damage, diagnosis or impairment)?

3. What is the probability for the injury to occur due to the reported trauma? (Is it biologically probable?)

4. What is the sensitivity of diagnostic testing used to determine the injury and is there clinical correlation with the symptoms (tissue damage, diagnosis and impairment)?

5. Is apportionment needed? (There must not be a more likely explanation for the symptoms)

6. Is there a valid permanent impairment present? (Based on the AMA Guides to the Evaluation of Permanent Impairment, 6th ed)

Judgments concerning causation should be based on scientific evidence and clinical rational. Once the diagnosis or impairment is determined the following is helpful to consider:

A CAUSAL RELATIONSHIP IS BIOLOGICALLY PLAUSIBLE WHEN (dependent on an accurate diagnosis and details of the trauma)
1. Is there a reasonable relationship between the injury (tissue damage / diagnosis) and trauma? (anatomically or physiologically possible)
2. Are the forces sufficient enough to cause the tissue damage or diagnosed condition in this occupant? (duration, intensity, or mechanism of exposure)
3. Is there evidence that traffic collisions are consistently or reliably associated with the claimed tissue damage, symptoms or diagnosis in peer-reviewed literature?
4. Is the cause and effect contiguous in time? (signs, symptoms or diagnosis should occur after the collision - temporal relationship)
5. Is there specificity in the association between the diagnosed conditions and trauma? (the absence of other factors)
Modified from American Medical Association: Disability Evaluation, second edition. Chicago, AMA 2003, page 96.

RISK FACTORS

A risk factor for an injury is any reason, characteristic, or exposure that increases the likelihood of developing a tissue damage or injury. In epidemiology, a risk factor is a variable associated with an increase in tissue damage or injury. The study of risk factors associated with traffic injuries is often complicated because of the numerous types of injuries reported, the inability to isolate variables, and the interconnected effect of multiple variables in combination at the same time.

A confounding factor is an independent risk factor for the outcome, and is also associated with the risk factor of acute or chronic pain following a traffic collision. Examples of possible acute confounding factors include age, gender, muscle type, body type, pre-collision physical and mental health, and severity and direction of crash impact. Because there are hundreds of different risk factors, each occupant has a different risk of injury.

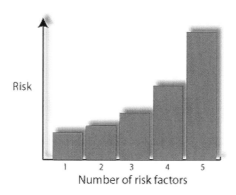

Risk

Number of risk factors

Cumulative risk states that the more factors, and the more intense the factors, then the greater the likelihood of developing symptoms. For example – Occupant #1, who has a history of previous neck surgery, gets hit from behind, which pushes her into the vehicle in front of her (second impact to the occupant), causing the air bags to deploy (third impact to the occupant). Occupant #2 also has a history of previous neck surgery but does not have a second or third impact. The cumulative risk factors increase the risk of injury to occupant #1 over occupant #2. Taking all the risk factors into consideration gives us the relative risk for each occupant.

Relative risk is the ratio of the probability of an event occurring (being injured) in an exposed group to the probability of the event occurring in a comparison, non-exposed group. The relative risk of each occupant takes into consideration the sum of the cumulative risk factors. Risk factors with independently low risk to causing acute injury can accumulate to cause a higher risk of acute injury. For traffic injuries, the risk factors for acute symptoms are different than the risk factors for chronic symptoms, but the cumulative and relative risk should still be analyzed.

Non-associated factors are factors identified as not being associated with the development of acute or chronic pain post-trauma. Correlation does not imply causation, or "with this, therefore because of this," means that having a trauma doesn't mean that symptoms will be present. Just because you are in a collision doesn't mean that you will have tissue damage or symptoms.

A coincidence is a series of events that happen at the same time and seem to have some connection but don't. This is very common in MRI or diagnostic testing findings which were present before the trauma but not identified until after the trauma.

ACUTE AND CHRONIC SYMPTOMS

In this section we will discuss risk factors for acute conditions and chronic conditions. **Surprisingly, many of the factors that have an influence on acute tissue damage are not prognostic of chronic symptoms.** The mechanism of acute pain (tissue damage) is not the same as the mechanism of chronic pain (destructive chronic damage). It's important to also realize that accuracy of the diagnosis and facts of the trauma are essential to evaluate.

As discussed in other chapters there is a vast difference between acute symptoms and chronic symptoms. Acute symptoms including pain are warning signs of tissue damage and typically lesion-based. Chronic symptoms including pain are signs of destructive changes in the brain, nervous system, or other biological tissue.

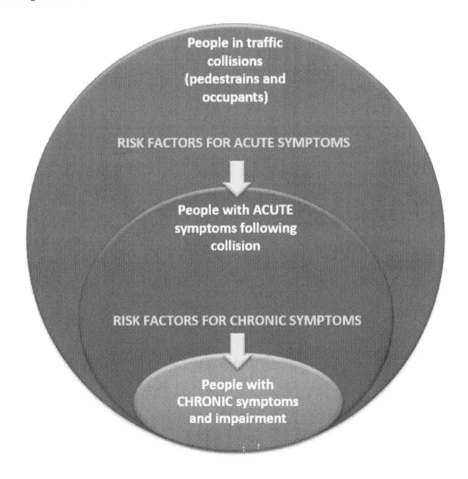

2 CATEGORIES OF RISK FACTORS FOR ACUTE SYMPTOMS

Based on scientific and medical literature, there are two major categories of factors that determine an occupant's risk for acute injury or tissue damage: human factors and collision factors. Some factors alone may not have a significant influence, yet when combined with other factors, they may increase the risk of acute injury. The graph below demonstrates that the more human factors or collision factors that an occupant has, the higher the relative risk of injury.

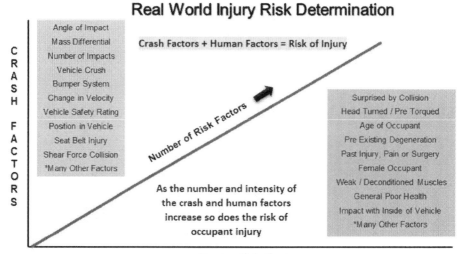

Analyzing the severity and number of risk factors gives valuable information to determine causation:

1. Human risk factors for acute injury: age, general health, diseases that slow healing, long thin neck, prior injuries, degenerative spine disease, history of pain before the accident, osteoporosis, diabetic, decreased muscle mass, and various other conditions that would be specific for the occupant. It must make clinical sense why a risk factor would increase the risk for injury.

2. Collision risk factors for acute injury (forces imposed on the occupant): vehicle specifics (size, weight, etc.), position in the car, type of bumper, distance from the head to the seat back, whether the occupant was surprised by the collision, the type of seatbelt used, angle of collision, whether the brakes were applied during collision, whether there were multiple collisions, and/or whether the occupant's head was turned during impact. There are many unique forces that can be imposed on an occupant.

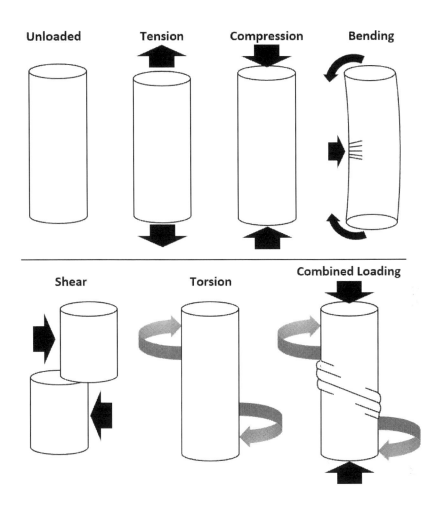

HUMAN RISK FACTORS FOR ACUTE SYMPTOMS

When considering acute injury causation and any subsequent post-traumatic symptoms or disorders, it is imperative for the provider and others to remember that there is no "typical" human in a crash environment.

Healthcare providers typically determine diagnosis, injury causation, and apportionment because of their knowledge and training in the human body and pathology. Anyone who believes that all persons act equally to varying environments, needs to look at prescribed medications and note how many different side effects can occur among the general population. If people vary in how they react to the same types of chemicals in a specific medication, the same differences must also be prevalent between humans in similar types of traumatic events, such as traffic collisions. There are several reasons why an individual can be different than what is generally representative of a group of subjects involved in a collision, including:

Gender
Although injury may occur to men and women, many studies show that women are 2-3 times as likely to experience an injury when involved in a collision. Females also have increased susceptibility for chronic symptoms once injured. Higher injury rates may be attributed to biomechanical, psychological, sociological, or anthropomorphic considerations.

Age
Injury may occur at any age, young or old. The likelihood of experiencing tissue damage following a traffic collision increases with age. As we reach middle age and beyond, our flexibility and strength gradually decline, the degenerative processes begin, and there is a longer history of pathology, all of which predispose the body to injury. In addition to longer recovery times and greater morbidity, injury susceptibility may also be greater in older occupants.

Prior Injury
Individuals who have had a prior injury or symptoms may be more likely to experience acute injury in a collision. Prior injuries may have a negative effect on the severity of the new injuries and tend to delay recovery time.

Acute on Chronic Conditions
Persons with past surgery, degeneration, bone spurs, stenosis or arthritis increases the risk of injury, pain, disability & new tissue damage. Degenerated or deconditioned joints, muscles, and ligaments have reduced tissue tensile strength, which increases the risk of acute tissue damage. Systemic arthritis, such as rheumatoid arthritis, lupus, psoriatic, and others, all increase the risk of pain and inflammation not just in joints, but in the entire body. Conditions such as osteoporosis and osteopenia can increase the risk of fractures during trauma.

There are 2 questions to ask when an acute injury or trauma overlays a chronic condition:
1. Was the preexisting condition dormant or symptomatic before the trauma?
2. Did the trauma cause a precipitation, recurrence, exacerbation, aggravation, or no change in the chronic condition?

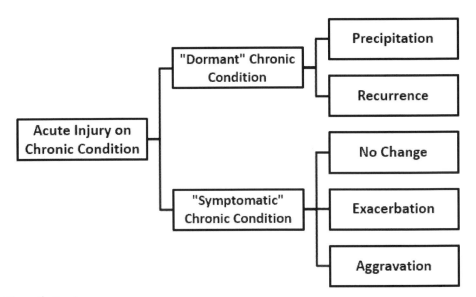

Genetic Factors

Research has shown that there is a genetic component to pain, pain processing, anxiety, tissue tensile strength, and other human factors that increase the risk of tissue damage and pain. Researchers from the University of North Carolina collected data from 838 patients who came to one of eight emergency departments in four states for care after a traffic collision. Clinical examination and blood test were performed. Findings revealed the FKBP5 gene variant was associated with a 20 percent higher risk of moderate to severe neck pain six weeks after a collision, as well as a greater extent of body pain.

Psychological Factors

Since anxiety is an important feature of traffic collisions and is known to influence the perception and experience of pain, post-traumatic stress symptoms may also alter the perception and experience of acute pain. There is consistent evidence that persons who report more frequent or more severe post-injury symptoms and greater pain intensity have a poorer prognosis for recovery from traffic injuries.

Anger and Blame

Getting into an "accident" is not fun. In many cases, the collision may have an external cause involving another person or persons. It can also be very difficult dealing with the insurance company, vehicle repair, doctors, family, and work. Feelings of stress or anger are often expressed in symptoms. Anger was found to be associated with physical and psychological complaints six months after a traffic collision. Research suggests that anger is an emotion that is associated with persistent symptoms and can influence the experienced pain.

Body Morphology
Different body types can have different risk factors for injury after trauma. A taller person can hit their head on the roof or knees on the dash. A smaller person may have to sit closer to the steering wheel and have an impact with the steering wheel. A thinner and less muscular neck can withstand less force than a short, thick neck. There are many possible morphological factors that can increase the risk of injury.

Coping
Coping can be defined as the way in which an individual behaviorally, cognitively, and emotionally adapts to manage external or internal stressors. Research has shown that an individual's coping style is an important moderator of the course of pain symptoms and the outcome of treatment. Negative expectations about the clinical course and prognosis could lead to a heightened pain experience, fear avoidance, or catastrophic interpretations of symptoms, thereby contributing to a bad prognosis. Patients who believe they can recover, who avoid catastrophizing about their condition, and who believe they are not severely disabled appear to function better than those who do not. Such beliefs may mediate some of the relationships between pain severity and fear avoidance.

COLLISION RISK FACTORS FOR ACUTE SYMPTOMS
There are literally hundreds of collision factors that can increase or decrease the risk of acute injury, but they must make clinical sense. Vehicle design, speed of operation, road design, road environment, driver skill, physical impairment, and driver behavior all contribute to the risk. Tissue damage to the human body occurs from external dynamic exposure to abnormal loads or motions that exceed physiological limits. Whether or not the forces are capable of causing acute tissue damage or injury depends largely on occupant factors. Vehicle crush, airbags, and seat belts are all essential safety and life saving features, but also may contribute to forces on the occupant.

When objects collide with each other, momentum changes. The vehicle being struck experiences an increase in its momentum, while the striking vehicle generally experiences a loss of momentum. There is an exchange of energy. Generally, this is known as conservation of momentum, which is an important concept in both accident reconstruction and injury causation analysis.

This information is provided to give you some general background in the forces involved in a collision. An injury causation analysis involves comparing the mechanical forces involved in the incident with the body's injury tolerance. For injury to occur, loads must be applied to tissue in a manner and with enough force to exceed the strength and tolerance of the tissue. The momentum is the mass (size) of the striking vehicle multiplied by the velocity (speed). Obviously, the heavier and faster the striking vehicle, the more force is involved. The angle of impact, amount of crush and any secondary impacts also factor in to the forces imposed on the occupants.

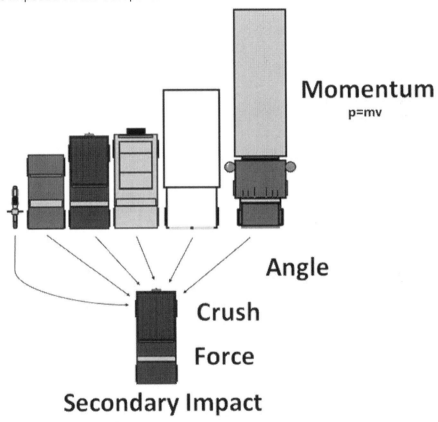

Momentum

p=mv

Angle

Crush

Force

Secondary Impact

Velocity Change (delta V)

The velocity change or acceleration-deceleration to the occupant is one of the most important collision factors for risk of injury. Acceleration refers to the change in velocity of a moving object within a certain period of time, either to a slower or faster pace, while deceleration exclusively refers to the negative acceleration (or slowing down) of an object.

Acceleration-deceleration of the brain occurs when the head is accelerated and then stopped suddenly. The change in velocity can traumatize the brain without the surface of the head ever contacting another object. In order to appreciate the potential complexities of acceleration-deceleration on the brain, it is important to have an understanding of the implications of these forces on the brain's mechanisms. We will discuss this in great detail later in the mechanism of injury chapter.

Often a defense engineer will estimate Delta V based on pictures of vehicle damage. The entire analysis is predicated on the assumption that scientists know how much Delta V is required to cause injury to all people and to each individual in particular. The truth is that insufficient testing has been performed to date on human volunteers to know how much force is required to cause injury to any particular individual.

Momentum

Generally; the larger the striking object, the more that object weighs, and the faster it's going, the more momentum it has. Being rear-ended by an 18-wheeler full of merchandise is different than being rear-ended by a motorcycle. Even low speed impacts and minor damage impacts with significant momentum can generate considerable forces and transfer energy to the occupant. These forces are often sufficient to cause varying degrees of bodily injury to high risk individuals. The amount of G force to which occupants of the vehicle are subject is one major factor relating to occupant injury.

Angle of Impact

The angle of the impact ultimately affects the angle of the forces on the occupant. Human connective tissue (including ligaments and tendons) exhibits both viscous and elastic properties when undergoing deformation. This is called viscoelasticity. Tension forces, compression forces, bending forces, shear forces, torque forces, and combined loading forces all can cause injury. Shear forces, torque forces, and combined loading forces typically cause more tissue damage because of the body's viscoelastic properties.

Vehicle crush

Crush or crumple zones are designed to absorb and redistribute the force of a collision. Crumple zones work by managing crash energy and absorbing it within the outer parts of the vehicle, rather than being directly transferred to the occupants. Crush, or vehicle damage, actually protects the occupant from external forces.

Bumper to Bumper Impact

If the bumper doesn't crush, as in low impact collisions, the people in the car absorb the energy. The purpose of having a bumper on your car is very specific. Many people think that its purpose is to prevent or lessen injury severity in a crash. In fact, bumpers are not considered safety features intended to protect occupants at all.

The purpose of bumpers is to reduce or prevent physical damage to the front and rear of vehicles in low-speed crashes. Bumpers are designed to minimize property damage due to bumper regulations by the National Highway Traffic Safety Administration ("NHTSA"). The NHTSA specifically says that car bumpers are "not a safety feature intended to prevent or mitigate injury severity to occupants in the passenger cars."

Trailer hitches

Trailer hitches and bumper on bumper impact may not result in much damage, but the transfer of energy is still present. The bumper is designed to prevent or reduce physical damage to the front and rear ends of passenger motor vehicles in low-speed collisions. Bumpers and trailer hitches are not a safety feature intended to prevent or mitigate injury severity to occupants in the passenger cars. Bumpers are designed to protect the hood, trunk, grille, fuel, exhaust, and cooling system, as well as safety related equipment such as parking lights, headlamps, and taillights, in low speed collisions. The NHTSA specifically states that car bumpers are "not a safety feature intended to prevent or mitigate injury severity to occupants in the passenger cars."

In a European study by Chalmers, with data from Folksam and Autoliv, they concluded that a vehicle equipped with a trailer hitch (tow bar) increases the risk of traffic injury by 22% if it is hit in the rear. Today, roughly 40% of the vehicles on the highway have receiver hitches. Although they are necessary for towing, they reduce rear end collision damage and INCREASE the risk of injury by creating a stiff "crash pulse". From an occupant's perspective, the crash pulse is the inertial event to which the vehicle's restraint systems must respond in order to mitigate the forces and accelerations that act on a passenger, and thus reduce injury risk.

Secondary Impacts

Secondary impacts with another external object or an object inside the vehicle complicate the dynamics of the force imposed on the occupant. Seatbelts and airbags are very effective at saving lives and should be worn at all times, but there is some evidence that they can actually cause minor injuries such as cuts, burns, and other minor injuries. The vehicle hitting a secondary impact such as a tree, wall, or another vehicle commonly imposes more forces on the occupant.

Body Position
An occupant's position may have an impact on the likelihood of experiencing injury. Tissue damage is more common when the body is twisted or turned, or if the person is leaning forward or in any other awkward position at the moment of impact.

Head Position
When the head is turned at the time of impact, asymmetric loads are placed on the spinal ligaments, facet joints, intervertebral discs, and spinal nerves. Additionally, having the head turned during a collision may increase the likelihood of more significant injuries to the cervical facet joints.

Surprise by the Collision
In many cases, drivers and passengers of vehicles that are struck from the rear have no warning of the impending collision. Preparedness for impact may reduce the risk of injury. Furthermore, since the neck is more vulnerable in the relaxed state, awareness plays a role in the severity of an injury, particularly ligament damage. Clinical studies have supported the assertion that if an occupant is aware of the impending impact, some preventive action can be taken to minimize injury risk. One study reported the risk of having chronic pain was 15 times greater when the occupant was unaware.

Front vs Rear Seating Location
Different seating locations within a vehicle may contribute to the likelihood of experiencing symptoms during a collision. A person occupying the front seat of an automobile has a higher risk of neck injury than passengers in the rear, possibly due to mechanical or head restraint differences.

Head Restraint
Incorrect adjustment of the restraint position may account for restraint ineffectiveness, and may actually increase injury. For a head restraint to properly protect passengers, it should be a placed at the center of gravity of the occupant's head, which is located approximately at the level of the top of a person's ears. If positioned lower, risk of neck injury may be greater. Peak facet-joint capsular strains were shown to occur prior to head restraint contact. Depending on an occupant's height, head restraint position and design may increase the likelihood of an injury, as some head restraints don't adequately protect tall occupants.

Rear Ended vs. Other Impacts

The point of impact is a factor in risk assessment of collisions. While large proportions of collisions involve frontal crashes, the risk of traffic injuries is higher in rear-impact collisions. One study found that individuals in rear-impact crashes are exposed to a more complex and unnatural neck movement upon being hit. They may experience a rapid change in direction of the head within a fraction of a second. Additionally, rear end collisions often cause the head to strike the head restraint, which may lead to further injury.

Impact with Vehicle of Greater Mass

The likelihood of experiencing injury may increase when a person has a collision with a vehicle larger than his or her own vehicle. In general, the relative mass between two colliding vehicles is an important determinant of the outcome of a collision. Since a vehicle with a larger mass transfers more energy to a smaller vehicle, injuries and symptoms may be more likely and more significant to occupants in the smaller vehicle.

RISK FACTORS FOR CHRONIC SYMPTOMS

While most people should expect to fully recover from acute traffic injuries within the first few months, approximately 25-50 percent of individuals injured in a traffic collision progress to long-term pain and chronic symptoms. Recovery after a traffic injury can typically be predicted with a high level of probability at six months post-collision.

The transition from acute to chronic pain following traffic collisions is a costly and growing problem. **Surprisingly, the bulk of evidence suggests that crash-related factors (e.g. impact direction, awareness of collision, head position) are NOT associated with the prognosis or development of chronic pain.** There is overwhelming evidence that biological, psychosocial, and neurological factors all play a role in the progression from acute pain to chronic pain. **Catastrophizing, stress response, pain and disability, irritability, neuropathic pain, and expectations (C-SPINE) are factors that have been shown to increase the risk of chronicity.**

C-SPINE

Regardless, from a management perspective, it's highly important to reduce the C-SPINE factors, pain, and symptoms as quickly as possible to minimize the progression to chronic pain. Other factors, such as genetics, functional testing, and neuropsychological evaluation may also have an influence on chronicity. Below are some other common factors associated with the development of chronic symptoms:

Valid Permanent Impairment
High Initial Pain Intensity
High Number of Different Symptoms
High Neck-Related Disability
Sensorimotor Dysfunction
High intensity headache
Radicular/Peripheral Neurological Symptoms
Cold Hypersensitivity/Hyperalgesia
Head Injury
Catastrophizing
Kinesiophobia
PTS

DEFINITIONS TO SUPPORT THIS CHAPTER

Human Factors - Variables such as physical makeup, health conditions, genetics, positional, psychosocial, and other factors that increase or decrease the risk of injury or disease during collision.

Collision Factors - Variables such as angle of impact, mass differential, number of impacts, vehicle crush, type of bumper system, vehicle safety rating, net change in velocity, position in vehicle, air bag impact, seat belt trauma, and other factors that increase or decrease the risk of injury or disease during collision.

Vehicle crush - Crush or crumple zones are designed to absorb and redistribute the force of a collision. Crumple zones work by managing crash energy, absorbing it within the outer parts of the vehicle, rather than being directly transferred to the occupants.

Newton's 1st Law of Motion - (Law of Inertia) An object at rest will stay at rest and an object in motion will stay in motion, unless acted upon by a net force.

Newton's 2nd Law of Motion - (Law of Acceleration) The acceleration of an object as produced by a net force is directly proportional to the magnitude of the net force, in the same direction as the net force, and inversely proportional to the mass of the object.

Newton's 3rd Law of Motion - For every action there is an equal and opposite reaction. According to Newton's 3rd Law, the forces they exert on each other must be equal and opposite.

Acceleration (a) - the rate of change of velocity; the rate at which an object speeds up.

Deceleration (d) - the opposite of acceleration; the rate at which an object slows down.

Acceleration-Deceleration - Cumulative force of a rapid acceleration followed by a rapid deceleration.

Velocity (v) - Speed with a directional component.

Force (F) - Force = Mass x Acceleration ($F = ma$)

Mass (m) - the quantity of matter in a body regardless of its volume or of any forces acting on it.

Momentum (p) - p=mv. The mass of an object multiplied by its velocity. It is a vectored quantity with both magnitude and direction.

The Law of Momentum Conservation - For a collision occurring between object 1 and object 2 in an isolated system, the total momentum of the two objects before the collision is equal to the total momentum of the two objects after the collision.

Impulse (J) - the product of force and time in which that force acts on an object.

Closing Speed - The speed differential between two vehicles traveling on the same line or the sum of the two speeds for opposing vehicles.

Conservation of Energy - The principle of physics that says the amount of energy in a closed system is constant regardless of the form of that energy.

Conservation of Momentum - The principle of physics that says the total momentum of two colliding bodies is equal before and after collision.

G-Force - A term used when accelerations are expressed as a multiple of the acceleration of gravity. The acceleration of gravity equaling 1G or 32.2 feet per second squared.

Viscoelasticity - Human connective tissue (including ligaments and tendons) exhibit both viscous and elastic properties when undergoing deformation.

Tension force - Pulling force transmitted axially.

Compression force - Axial or inward ("pushing") forces.

Bending force - Tensile and compressive stresses increase proportionally with bending moment.

Shear force - Unaligned forces pushing one part of a body in one specific direction, and another part of the body in the opposite direction.

Torque force - A twisting or torsion force that tends to cause rotation.

Combined loading force - Any mixture of any compressive, shear, tension, torque or bending forces. This force is the most damaging to the discs, joints, muscles and ligaments.

FURTHER READING TO SUPPORT THIS CHAPTER

Biomechanics of Musculoskeletal Injury, Second Edition : Whiting PhD, Zernicke PhD, March 17, 2008

Whiplash and Mild Traumatic Brain Injury, Arthur C. Croft , Spine Research Institute of Sa; 1st edition (2009)

Whiplash-Associated Diseases, American Medical Association, , Rene Cailliet, 2007

Motor Vehicle Collision Injuries, Second Ed, Lawrence Nordhoff, Jones & Bartlett Publishers 2005

Whiplash: evidence base for clinical practice, Michele Sterling PhD, Churchill Livingstone, 2011

"The Anatomy & Biomechanics of Acute and Chronic Whiplash Injury", Traffic Injury Prevention, 10: 2, 101-112

Malcolm C. Robbins (1997) Society of Automobile Engineers "Lack of relationship between vehicle damage and occupant injury." 97-02-01: (#970494): 117-9

Foreman SM, Croft AC: Whiplash Injuries: The Cervical Acceleration/Deceleration Syndrome (ed 3). Baltimore, Lippincott Williams & Wilkins Co., 2002.

Carroll LJ, Holm LW, Hogg-Johnson S, Cassidy JD, Haldeman S, et al. Course and prognostic factors for neck pain in whiplash-associated disorders (WAD). Results of the bone and joint decade 2000–2010 task force on neck pain and its associated disorders. Eur Spine J 2008;17(Suppl 1):83–92

CHAPTER 4
DIAGNOSIS AND TISSUE DAMAGE
A good diagnosis is the first step to a successful treatment.
Tissue damage typically heals in a predictable timeframe.
There is not always a relationship between tissue damage and pain perception.
If you hurt your back and get an early MRI, you've reduced your chances of recovery.

SUMMARY – Determining the extent of tissue damage and primary cause of pain in a traffic collision is important to ensure a successful treatment outcome. Differentiating incidental pathologies from new tissue damage pathologies is vital to prevent chronic pain and have realistic expectations. Pain and other symptoms can derive from many potential anatomic sources, such as nerve roots, muscle, fascial structures, bones, joints, intervertebral discs (IVDs), and organs within the abdominal cavity. Additionally, symptoms can be caused by or amplified as a consequence of abnormal neurological processing. There is a multifactorial intertwining of social, psychological, biological, and structural components to acute and chronic pain.

Determining the severity of anatomical tissue damage is essential and potentially lifesaving. Visceral, vascular, and/or cancer pain are rare, but need to be screened for in all cases. Acute nociceptive (tissue damage) pain represents the normal response to chemical irritation, noxious assault, or injury of tissues such as skin, vascular system, nerves, muscles, visceral organs, joints, tendons, ligaments, or bones.

Visceral pain can be caused by injury, inflammation, or trauma to the internal organs. Visceral pain is also caused by obstruction of visceral tubes and lack of blood supply (ischemic) to viscera. Visceral tissues are stomach, intestine, appendix, lungs, heart, gall bladder, ureter, kidney, urinary bladder, spleen, uterus, and pancreas.

Vascular pain develops when there is pathology to the vascular system or interruption in blood flow to a tissue, organ or nerves. Examples include: Vasculitis (inflammation of blood vessels), coronary artery disease, circulatory problems, vascular ruptures (breakages), constrictions, blood vessel spasms, ischemia, peripheral vascular disease, or trauma injuries (including accidents, stab wounds, and gunshot wounds).

Cancer pain has many different causes and different types. Most cancer pain is caused by the tumor irritation or pressing on bones, nerves, or other organs in the body. Sometimes the pain is caused by cancer treatment. The pain can also be from the cancer itself growing into or destroying nearby tissue. The tumor can also release chemicals that can cause pain.

Red Flags are warning signs and symptoms that indicate more serious or potentially life-threatening conditions. These "red flags" include but are not limited to: history of blunt trauma, fever, incontinence, bleeding, unexplained weight loss, history of cancer, severe tissue damage, numbness, drug abuse, loss of consciousness, slurred speech, vision problems, paresthesia, drop foot, intense unrelenting pain, and blood in the urine. Conditions such as severe spinal fractures, severe dislocation, severe ligament damage, nerve damage, visceral, vascular, cancer, permanent impairments, and other potentially life-threatening conditions are also considered red flags.

Yellow flags are warning signs and symptoms that are recognized as having an influence on long term disease outcomes, which may complicate assessment and treatment. Yellow flags are factors or conditions suggesting an increased risk of progression to long-term distress, disability, and potential drug misuse. They include the patient's attitudes, beliefs, emotions, behaviors, and family and/or workplace factors. Conditions such as spinal fractures, cervical disc herniation, dislocation, severe ligament damage, brain injury, post-surgical pain, and other more significant tissue damage are also factors.

Considerations when diagnosing pain:
- Body Region (e.g.: neck, back, head, abdomen, etc.)
- Body Systems (e.g.: cardiovascular, nervous, musculoskeletal, digestive, endocrine, etc.)
- Characteristics of Pain (e.g.: sharp, burning, ache, dull, shooting, etc.)
- Pain Intensity (e.g.: severe, moderate, mild)
- Pain Frequency (e.g.: constant, frequent, occasional, on & off, etc.)
- Time since onset of pain (e.g.: hours, days, months, years, etc.)
- Etiology (e.g.: trauma, degenerative, congenital, infective, psychological, etc.)

Some symptoms after an injury are normal physiological responses to tissue damage. It's important to stop thinking that every minor symptom or pain requires a diagnosis, testing or treatment. In some cases, focusing on incidental findings on MRI can lead to catastrophizing or fear avoidance.

In cases where the tissue damage or potential for tissue damage is very minor and the reported symptoms are severe, the clinician needs to look for other causes of the symptoms. Malingering, amplification, apportionment, factitious disorder, and somatization should be evaluated for in these cases.

AN ACCURATE DIAGNOSIS

"A good diagnosis is the first step to a successful treatment". A good diagnosis starts with comprehensive workup and examination with clinical correlation of the findings. Determining the extent of anatomical tissue damage is essential in a traffic injury case. The reporting of pain alone is not enough to justify prolonged care.

The wrong diagnosis often results in unsuccessful treatment and can be potentially dangerous. Furthermore, a therapeutic approach geared towards controlling the symptoms (pain) rather than fixing the pain generator is also usually unproductive long term. Appropriate care is best achieved with the combination of an accurate diagnosis, a proper treatment plan, and patient selection.

The provider also has a significant influence on the quality of the diagnosis. Diagnosing pain by the type of pain and then by the anatomical pain generator are essential first steps in effective patient selection for treatment. This chapter will go over the methodology for an accurate diagnosis and patient selection.

METHODOLOGY FOR A DIAGNOSIS

A diagnosis is only as accurate as the information provided by physical findings and the examiner. The following is a brief overview for the framework for an accurate diagnosis.

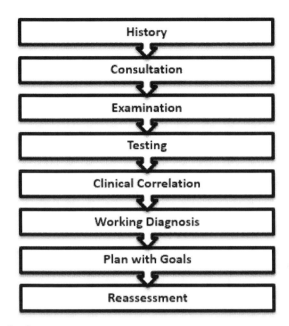

History (Subjective)

The history is reported by the patient and comprises of complete reporting of the current and past health history. A detailed history is essential in obtaining an accurate diagnosis. The history is the first component of an accurate diagnosis. Details such as the relationship of symptoms to activity, the frequency of symptoms, and the location of symptoms help to focus the diagnosis. A useful and often overlooked tool in obtaining the history is to have the patient localize the area of pain by simply pointing to the symptomatic region.

Pain drawings and questionnaires concerning the reported symptoms are helpful. The PQRSTU acronym is a great format to follow:

- Present and Past Pain / Symptoms (history of trauma, surgery, illness or similar symptoms in the past)
- Quality of Pain
- Region of Pain and or Radiation
- Severity of Symptoms
- Timing (onset, duration)
- U (How the pain or symptoms effect You / the patient)

Pain History: A Systematic Approach Using PQRSTU Acronym

Past & Present

- Provocation: What happened? What elicits pain or aggravates it/makes it worse?
- Palliation: What makes it better? What has been tried? Include both pharmacological (over the

65

counter and prescription) and non-pharmacological (e.g., ice/heat, massage, acupuncture, chiropractic, physical therapy, meditation)? Response to treatment: How well did each treatment work? Any adverse effects?

- Past: Surgeries, conditions, diseases, and past history of present problem.

Quality of Pain.

For example: is the pain sharp or dull, throbbing?

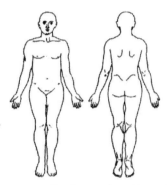

Region of Pain/Radiation.

- Region or location of pain
- Radiation of pain

Severity of Pain.

Numeric pain intensity scale:
- Asks the patient to rate their pain intensity on a scale of 0 to 10
- Visual analogue rating scales

Timing.

Questions about time and pain including the following:
- Onset: When did the pain start? Is the pain immediate or delayed?
- How long after precipitating factors does it start?
- Time of day: When does the pain occur?

- Pattern: Is it intermittent or constant pain?
- Duration: How long does the pain last?

U (How it affects you).

Assessment of functioning is critical in determining the extent of treatment needed.
- Patients' mood, work/activities, relationships, etc, may be affected by pain
- Start with Activities of Daily Living assessment
- Supplement with open-ended questions regarding pain effects on functioning

Clinical Consultation

The consultation is where the provider discusses in more detail the reported symptoms and history. This is also where the provider looks for red and yellow flags, or other signs of severe pathology. The extent of the consultation depends on the present ailment, review of systems, past, family and/or social history, and the nature of the presenting problem(s). The patient consultation provides enough information to start forming ideas about a possible diagnosis or at least a diagnostic category.

Consultation tips:
- Communicate openly with good eye contact; be straightforward; listen and ask questions.
- Elicit patient's perceptions of the pain and associated feelings and expectations.
- Ask non-leading, open ended questions to gather information at first.
- Draw the patient out, when appropriate ("Can you say more about...").
- Ask detailed questions about the trauma or triggering event.
- Be present to nonverbal cues of pain and dysfunction.
- Listen for possibly life-threatening conditions, such as referred pain from viscera, blood vessels, peripheral vascular disease, thromboembolism, and cancer.
- Ask questions about past history of cancer, surgery, psychosocial, or similar conditions.

Examination (Objective Signs)

The areas and extent of physical examination is based on the information gathered in the history and consultation. This includes physical inspection, observation of gait, palpation, movement, orthopedic testing, neurological testing, strength testing, and other condition-specific procedures. Because musculoskeletal symptoms can be the result of orthopedic, neurologic, or rheumatologic processes, a comprehensive neuromuscular examination should incorporate a detailed neurologic and musculoskeletal examination. Observation of objective findings or signs aids in narrowing the diagnosis.

Diagnostic Testing
For most acute musculoskeletal conditions, imaging or testing is generally not indicated or required. Imaging should be reserved for patients who reveal suspicious findings on history or examination. Under certain circumstances, however, imaging may be ordered to rule out specific causes of pain, including fracture, dislocation, tumors, and spinal stenosis. Imaging and other types of tests include:

X-ray is often the first imaging technique used to look for broken bones or an injured vertebra. X-rays show the bony structures and any vertebral misalignment or fractures. Soft tissue injuries to the muscles, ligaments, or discs are not visible on conventional x-rays. In fact, most injuries do not show on x-rays. "It is of little value to perform flexion and extension studies when generalized muscle spasm is present following acute trauma." *Motor Vehicle Collision Injuries (page 147). Motor Vehicle Collision Injuries, Second Ed, Lawrence Nordhoff, Jones & Bartlett Publishers 2005.*

Functional or Motion X-ray is a radiology procedure to see the function of joints and ligaments. While the ligaments themselves are not shown on the x-ray images, the effect of injured ligaments can be ascertained by abnormal movement of the spinal vertebral bodies in relation to each other. An analogy is to watch leaves blowing in a tree, where we cannot see the wind, but we can see the effect of the wind. Likewise, even though we cannot see the cervical ligaments, we can see the results of ligamentous injuries by abnormal movement of the vertebral bodies and facet joints, which is easily observed by anyone trained in musculoskeletal radiology using standard radiology practices. This is not performed in the acute stage of care.

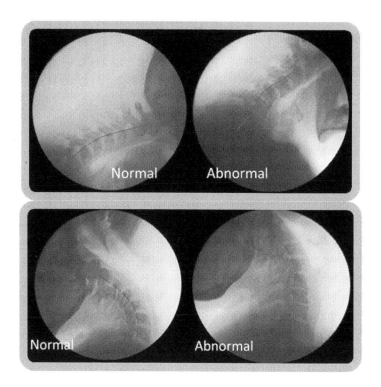

Normal   Abnormal

Normal   Abnormal

Computerized tomography (CT) is used to see spinal structures that cannot be seen on conventional x-rays, such as fracture, spinal stenosis, or tumors. Using a computer, the CT scan creates a three-dimensional image from a series of two dimensional pictures.

BrainScope is an acute brain injury assessment device that uses revolutionary EEG-based technology that facilitates confident decision-making on the spot. BrainScope One system (FDA-cleared as Ahead 300[1]) is an easy-to-use, non-invasive, hand-held platform that empowers physicians to make more accurate head injury assessments quickly at the point-of-care. It's important to differentiate between mTBI, PTSD, mental health issues and catastrophizing.

Magnetic resonance imaging (MRI) uses a magnetic force instead of radiation to create a computer-generated image. Unlike x-ray, which shows only bony structures, MRI scans also produce images of soft tissues such as muscles, ligaments, tendons, and blood vessels. An MRI may be ordered if a problem such as infection, tumor, inflammation, disc herniation, or if pressure on a nerve is suspected. MRI is a noninvasive way to identify a condition requiring prompt surgical treatment. Although disc pathology seems to be one possible contributing factor in the development of chronic symptoms after injury, it may be unnecessary to examine these patients in the acute phase with magnetic resonance imaging; correlating initial symptoms and signs to magnetic resonance imaging findings is difficult because of the relatively high proportion of false-positive results. Magnetic resonance imaging is indicated later in the course of treatment in patients with persistent arm pain, neurologic deficits, or clinical signs of nerve root compression, to diagnose disc herniations requiring surgery.

MRI is not the answer to a diagnosis in the vast majority of patients developing long-lasting pain after a traffic injury. Early MRI scans do not predict prognosis. It may be relevant to focus future trials upon imaging of the upper cervical spine, including functional imaging. *Are early MRI findings correlated with long-lasting symptoms following whiplash injury? A prospective trial with 1-year follow-up, Eur Spine J (2008) 17:996–1005*

Electrodiagnostics are procedures that, in the setting of low back pain, are primarily used to confirm whether a person has lumbar radiculopathy. The procedures include electromyography (EMG), nerve conduction studies (NCS), and evoked potential (EP) studies. EMG assesses the electrical activity in a muscle and can detect if muscle weakness results from a problem with the nerves that control the muscles. Very fine needles are inserted in muscles to measure electrical activity transmitted from the brain or spinal cord to a particular area of the body.

NCSs are often performed along with EMG to exclude conditions that can mimic radiculopathy. In NCSs, two sets of electrodes are placed on the skin over the muscles. The first set provides a mild shock to stimulate the nerve that runs to a particular muscle. The second set records the nerve's electrical signals, and from this information nerve damage that slows conduction of the nerve signal can be detected. EP tests also involve two sets of electrodes – one set to stimulate a sensory nerve, and the other placed on the scalp to record the speed of nerve signal transmissions to the brain.

Facet Joint Diagnostic Blocks are performed with the anticipation that if successful, treatment may proceed to facet neurotomy at the diagnosed levels (a procedure that is considered "under study"). Therapeutic intra-articular and medial branch blocks are typically not recommended.

Clinical Correlation (Decision Making)
This is when the signs, symptoms, history, consultation, exam findings, orthopedic testing, and diagnostic testing are in general agreement with a

possible diagnosis. If there is no correlation then further testing is required. It is also important to determine if there are any contraindications to possible treatments.

Working diagnosis
The working diagnosis is the highest diagnosis on the list of the possible diagnoses, or the most likely diagnosis based on the information provided. It guides future diagnostic tests and treatment. A working diagnosis of the underlying pain condition is established based on putting together all information so far: signs, symptoms, history, physical examination, and diagnostic testing results currently available. The working diagnosis is updated on future visits or on reevaluations.

Plan with goals
Every good treatment plan starts with a clear goal (or set of goals). Having a clear measurable goal makes sure everyone is on the same page and keeps you both accountable to focusing on what is necessary. The treatment plan then follows up with how each party will work to achieve the goal(s). This includes home care, avoidance of triggering, and delay in healing factors. Given the challenges of chronic musculoskeletal pain and disability, establishing a clear prognosis in the acute stage has become increasingly recognized as a valuable approach to mitigate chronic problems.

Reassessment
At sent time frames, usually every 4-6 weeks, it is essential to reevaluate the symptoms, response to care, and diagnosis. If the patient is not improving, the diagnosis needs to be re assessed. If the patient is improving as expected, a new set of goals for continued improvement are needed.

CLASSIFYING PAIN BY TYPE OF PAIN
At the highest level, pain can be divided into 3 categories: acute pain, chronic pain, or acute on chronic pain. Diagnosing the anatomical cause of pain involves first putting it into these broad categories and then working toward more specific anatomical diagnosis. This information is gathered during the history, consultation, examination, and any testing.

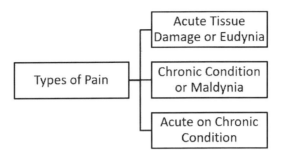

Diagnosis of Acute (Eudynia / Tissue damage) Pain

With acute pain, there is usually underlying tissue damage that accompanies the pain, such as a broken bone (somatic pain), ovarian cyst (visceral pain), strain injury (somatic pain), kidney stone (visceral pain), blood clot (vascular pain), nerve compression from a herniated disc (neuropathic pain), or cancer pain. Any possible life-threatening condition or severe pathology needs to be screened first. Acute pain is a type of pain that typically lasts less than 3 to 6 months.

Acute musculoskeletal pain involves the activation of pain receptors in muscles, ligaments, or joint capsules. This is often referred to as nociception pain. Pain after trauma or injury is usually attributed to strains of muscles or sprains of ligaments. Pain from a muscle or ligament can be referred to the joint on which that muscle operates, or ligament supports. Pain reported over a joint, therefore, does not necessarily imply a source of pathology is in that joint. The source may be in one of the nearby muscles or ligaments.

The cardinal clinical features are pain, tenderness, and impaired range of movement. In cases with a recent history of injury, swelling is also distinguishing sign of injury.

Diagnosis of Chronic (Maldynia / Destructive) Pain

Destructive tissue damage or an underlying condition may be found in a patient with chronic pain, but sometimes an exact cause of the symptoms cannot be determined. Chronic pain has been recognized as pain that persists past normal healing time and, hence, lacks the acute warning function of physiological nociception. Chronic symptoms are usually progressive and may involve multiple body systems. Chronic pain is typically any pain that lasts for more than three months and persists after injuries heal for no apparent biological cause.

Common categories of chronic pain include the following:
- Neuropathic (e.g., phantom limb pain, CRIPS)
- Peripheral Nerve Entrapment (e.g., carpel tunnel, piriformis syndrome)

- Muscle pain (e.g., atrophy, past injury)
- Inflammatory (e.g., RA, Lupus, infection)
- Degenerative (e.g., low back pain due to OA)
- Visceral (e.g., hepatitis, COPD)
- Metabolic (e.g., diabetes, gout)
- Vascular (e.g., heart disease, stroke)
- Neuropathic & Muscle pain (e.g., fibromyalgia)
- Cancer pain (depends on tissue and type of cancer)
- Postsurgical pain (depends on surgery)

Diagnosis of Acute on Chronic Condition

As the name implies, this is when an acute injury (usually a trauma) occurs on top of a chronic condition. This is very common, but not usually addressed. Examples of chronic conditions that can be made symptomatic after trauma are: lupus, stenosis, degeneration, deconditioning, arthritis, past surgery, RA, PTSD, and many other conditions.

The phrase "preexisting" or "chronic" often causes confusion, but there are only two main types of chronic conditions. The first type is known as "inactive" or "dormant," where there is no evidence that a pre-existing condition was causing pain or symptoms before the acute event. The second type is known as an "active" or "symptomatic". This is when there is evidence that a pre-existing condition was causing pain or symptoms before the acute event. The difference between a dormant vs. symptomatic preexisting conditions (no pain vs pain) is "like night and day."

The process of differentiating dormant vs. symptomatic is called apportionment. Apportionment is an allocation of causation among multiple factors that caused or significantly contributed to the injury or disease and resulting impairment. When the chronic condition is dormant before the trauma (not causing any pain or symptoms), it is important to differentiate if this is a precipitation or a recurrence. Conversely, when the chronic condition is symptomatic before the trauma (pain or symptoms were present), it is important to differentiate if this is an aggravation or an exacerbation. This may not be known entirely until the end of treatment.

There are 2 questions to ask when an acute injury or trauma overlays a chronic condition:

1. Was the preexisting condition dormant or symptomatic before the trauma?
2. Did the trauma cause a precipitation, recurrence, exacerbation, aggravation or no change in the chronic condition?

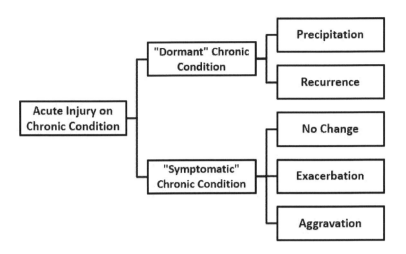

Combinations of direct trauma and a preexisting disease process are more difficult to assess for causality and apportionment. One must determine if the requirements of temporal relationship, biologic plausibility, literature support, and sufficient injury have been met. American Medical Association: Disability Evaluation, second edition. Chicago, AMA 2003, page 99 -100.

APPORTIONMENT DEFINITIONS	
Precipitation	Trauma caused a new condition for which the claimant was at risk for but may have never developed.
Recurrence	Reappearance of signs and symptoms attributed to a prior condition.
Aggravation	A permanent worsening of a prior condition.
Exacerbation	A temporary worsening of a prior condition. The condition is expected to return to a baseline.
Acceleration	Speeds the course of the disease, which would have become symptomatic, was more rapid due to injury. Disease not worse than it would be without the trauma just occurs sooner.
American Medical Association: Disability Evaluation, second edition. Chicago, AMA 2003, page 99 -100.	

Pain after an Injury

The process of determining the cause of pain after an injury is the same for pain in general, but more emphasis is put on the extent of acute tissue damage, causation, and apportionment. Chronic pain is usually initially only discussed to determine pre-trauma status.

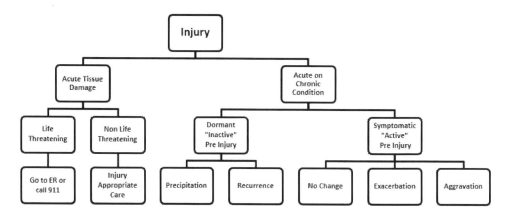

Once "dormant" or "symptomatic" chronic condition status is determined, it's important to evaluate if an exacerbation, aggravation, precipitation, or recurrence occurred. At a later date, both "dormant" and "symptomatic" conditions will be evaluated to determine if an acceleration has occurred. It's also important to determine if the injury will accelerate the degenerative process.

DIAGNOSIS BY PAIN GENERATOR

Narrowing down a diagnosis to the pain generator requires the provider to be a good detective. Each anatomical structure has a different pain profile, and it is common that more than one pain generator can be causing pain at the same time. In traffic injuries, this process helps to determine the nature of tissue damage. The table below outlines common findings in each pain generator by anatomical class:

Pain Type	Sclerotome (Somatic)	Dermatomal	Myofascial	Viscerogenic	Neurogenic	Psychogenic
Primary pain generators	Facet joint ligaments, deep muscles, outer disc, periosteum, uncovertebral joint, nerve roots & dura	Compression or irritation of the dorsal root ganglia	Myofascial and connective tissue	Visceral (organs) or vascular tissue	Central nervous system or peripheral nervous system	Cerebral cortex or patient induced
Common description of pain	General dull ache pain, sharp localized pain over joint, stiff, HA, sclerodermal referred pain	Sharp shooting pain, radiates in dermatomal pattern, paresthesia	Localized burning pain, dull ache that refers pain from TP, tightness	Deep, sharp, pressure, crushing, tearing, burning, throbbing	Burning, skin crawling, crushing, tingling, & hypersensitivity	Poorly defined, general pain with variable pattern
Physical findings	Mechanical stress & motion causes pain, patient often has limited range of motion / stiffness	Orthopedic & neurological signs / tests, atrophy, sensory & motor changes	Trigger point (TP) and/or referred pain on palpating muscle	Signs of distress, pain not relieved by rest or typical procedures	Allodynia, hyperalgesia, sympathetic symptoms, poor motor control, hypoesthesia	None or findings may not make clinical sense
Common disorders	Facet joint syndrome, internal disc derangement, arthritis, fracture, joint dysfunction, subluxation, sprain, adhesions	Herniated disc, canal stenosis, trauma, or space-occupying lesions	Levator scapulae, trapezius suboccipital, splenius capitis, SCM, & fibro-myalgia	Visceral or vascular	Peripheral nerve entrapments, neuropathies, tumors, MS, myelopathy RSD, & shingles	Mental illness, depression, malingering
Further diagnostic testing	Functional x-ray, diagnostic joint injection, CT	MRI, nerve testing	Clinical findings of TP and injections	Diagnostic specific for pathology	MRI, nerve testing	Psychiatric workup
Common coexisting findings	Myofascial	Sclerotome & myofascial	Sclerotome	Myofascial	Myofascial, Sclerotome, & dermatomal	Viscerogenic & myofascial
Condition progresses to	Dermatomal and/or neurogenic	Neurogenic	Sclerotome and/or neurogenic	Visceral or vascular failure	Loss or altered neurological functioning & neuroplasticity	Neurosis

Each of the tissue types described above could be injured if the trauma-induced forces exceed that tissue's tolerance. Anatomically, muscles and ligaments are commonly damaged, and are a common cause of pain in many traffic collisions. The brain, bones, disc, facet joints, skin, face, and organs are infrequently damaged during traffic collisions but, if damaged, are typically more severe tissue damage injuries. Early improvement of tissue healing helps to prevent worsening of tissue damage and avoid chronicity.

There is evidence supporting a lesion-based model in acute and chronic traffic injuries, but it's also important to remember that lack of macroscopically identifiable tissue damage does not rule out the presence of painful lesions. Below are a few pathoanatomical tissue damage lesions commonly found in traffic collisions:

1. Muscles
2. Ligaments
3. Facet joints and capsular ligament (Zygapophyseal Joints)
4. Dorsal root ganglion (DRG) and Nerve Roots
5. Intervertebral disc
6. Head injury (concussions)
7. PTSD
8. Dislocations
9. Bones (fractures)
10. Visceral or vascular

IMPAIRMENT

The American Medical Association: Guides to the Evaluation of Permanent Impairment is a book used by doctors and others to assign percentage ratings to those who have suffered injuries. The rating system described by the Guides has been under development since 1958, with the latest edition (the 6th edition) being published in 2007. **The American Medical Association: Guides to the Evaluation of Permanent Impairment is the "gold standard" for determining serious injury and impairment.**

The AMA Guides to the Evaluation of Permanent Impairment was assembled in response to the need for a standardized, objective rating system which would describe the amount of damage caused by various injuries and illnesses. The rating systems described in the AMA Guides to the Evaluation of Permanent Impairment were developed by committees of experts. The ratings described by the Guides have been adopted by workers compensation and injury compensation systems in most states of the United States and a number of other countries.

As traditionally used, *impairment* refers to a problem with a structure or organ of the body, *disability* is a functional limitation with regard to a particular activity, and *handicap* refers to a disadvantage in filling a role in life relative to a peer group. The beauty of an impairment rating is that if the clinical findings are fully described, any knowledgeable observer may check the findings with the

Guides criteria. Any other observer or physician following the methods in the Guides to evaluate the same patient should report similar findings.

Impairment is a significant deviation, loss or loss of use of any body structure or function in an individual with a health condition, disorder or disease. An anatomical, physiological, or psychological abnormality that can be shown by medically acceptable clinical and laboratory diagnostic techniques with clinical correlation.

TRAFFIC INJURY GUIDELINES

There are many publications, articles, and guidelines for treatment and care of traffic injuries: Croft Guidelines, Quebec Task Force Guidelines, Official Disability Guidelines, Canadian Guidelines, Australian Whiplash Guidelines, ACOEM Guidelines, Physical Therapy Guidelines, Chiropractic Guidelines, Diagnostic Testing Guidelines, Medical Treatment Guidelines, Internal Insurance Guidelines, Impairment Guidelines, and more. These publications are guidelines, not inflexible proscriptions, and they should not be used as sole evidence for an absolute standard of care.

Guidelines can assist clinicians in making decisions for specific conditions and help payors make reimbursement determinations, but they cannot consider the uniqueness of each patient's clinical circumstances. In cases where the care or testing is an exception to guidelines, the provider should document:
1. Extenuating circumstances of the case that warrant performance of the treatment, including the rationale for procedures.
2. Patient co-morbidities.
3. Objective signs of functional improvement for treatment conducted thus far.
4. Measurable goals and progress points expected from additional treatment.
5. Additional evidence that supports the health care provider's case.

TRAFFIC INJURY TREATMENT BEST PRACTICES AND EVIDENCED BASED CARE

Best practices and evidenced based care integrate three basic principles: (1) the best available research evidence bearing on whether and why a treatment works; (2) clinical expertise (clinical judgment and experience), to rapidly identify each patient's unique health state and diagnosis, their individual risks, and the benefits of potential interventions; and (3) patient preferences and values. This is a way of providing health care that is guided by a thoughtful integration of the best available scientific knowledge with clinical expertise. This approach allows the practitioner to critically assess research data, clinical guidelines, and other information resources in order to correctly identify the clinical problem, apply the most high-quality intervention, and re-evaluate the outcome for future improvement.

Evidence based care contains three elements: research, clinical judgment, and patient values. Best practices are clinical judgments regarding patient care that are informed by the best evidence and balanced by patient complexity and provider experience to improve the quality and reduce the costs of care. The clinical decision-making is according to evidence-based research. However, it is also outcome-based, encouraging innovation for the future of health care delivery.

When a provider determines that prolonged or continued treatment is indicated within an episode of care, the following criteria are necessary: (1) There is a reasonable expectation for improvement or the patient is demonstrating a reasonable rate of improvement. A reasonable rate of improvement would be influenced by condition chronicity, patient age, co-morbid factors, frequency of care, and exposure to activities that would impede progress. (2) If sufficient evidence exists demonstrating that reduction or withdrawal of care has and will continue to have a deleterious effect on the patient.

OFFICIAL DISABILITY GUIDELINES (ODG)

I often utilize the Official Disability Guidelines because they are evidence-based guidelines. ODG is designed for clinical practice as well as utilization review/management. Evidence-based research provides the basis for sound clinical practice guidelines and recommendations. The overall objectives are:

- To improve outcomes and patient satisfaction by focusing on restoration of functional capacity through prompt, responsible delivery of healthcare based on the best evidence.
- To reduce excessive utilization of services (and corresponding medical costs).
- To identify and target ineffective and harmful procedures, thus reducing risk on the injured.
- To improve clinical practice/utilization management by indexing procedures adjacent to a summary of their effectiveness based on supporting evidence, provided by way of link, in abstract form.
- To automate approval for universally effective treatment methods where appropriate, reducing friction and administrative delays on necessary medical care.
- To help the injured get back to work in good time, safely, easily, and effectively.

- To take evidence-based medicine to its logical endpoint – the convergence of health, wellness, productivity, efficiency, and responsible, cost-effective medical care.

The ODG acknowledges that they, "are guidelines, not inflexible proscriptions, and they should not be used as sole evidence for an absolute standard of care." ODG is a good mix of an immense guideline and evidence-based research.

INCIDENTAL FINDINGS

It's extremely important to differentiate the pain generator from any incidental but dormant pathology, such as degenerative disc disease or disc bulging. I have seen many cases where the patient underwent spine surgery, and surgery was not successful because the pain generator was not the area operated on. Over the years, a few patients made it to me before surgery, and we were able to help them without surgery.

A few years ago, a patient came for treatment related to an auto collision. I diagnosed him with a strain sprain injury and said that he should get better in 4-6 weeks. He already had an appointment with his PCP scheduled for a yearly physical the next day and I said that it was good that he still gets his yearly physical. Upon return to my office the patient stated that his PCP agreed with my diagnosis but that after running blood tests that he also has diabetes. My patient asked if diabetes could be from the accident because he never was diagnosed with diabetes before but was borderline for many years. I stated that the diabetes takes years to form and is due to lifestyle and not the collision. This is a great example of an incidental finding.

We love imaging so much in western medicine that we spend about $15 billion worth in it each year. Although imaging can give a fantastic insight into pathology, it doesn't come without its own negative side effects. For example, studies have shown that early MRI's performed on individuals with low back pain can lead to inferior outcomes, possibly due to the threatening language, negative self-perception, and nocebo that may come with it. In fact, I have seen cases where the MRI findings induced pain, disability, and even radiculopathy. Below are some common incidental findings in different areas of the body:

Cervical Spine

Disc bulging was frequently observed in asymptomatic subjects, even including those in their 20s. The number of patients with minor disc bulging increased from age 20 to 50 years. Most subjects presented with disc bulging (87.6%), which significantly increased with age in terms of frequency, severity, and number of levels. Even most subjects in their 20s had bulging discs, with 73.3% and 78.0% of males and females, respectively. In contrast, few asymptomatic subjects were diagnosed with spinal cord compression (SCC), (5.3%) or increased signal intensity (2.3%). These numbers increased with age, particularly after age 50 years. SCC mainly involved 1 level (58%) or 2 levels (38%), and predominantly occurred at C5–C6 (41%) and C6–C7 (27%). Spine: 15 March 2015 - Volume 40 - Issue 6 - p 392–398. Abnormal Findings on Magnetic Resonance Images of the Cervical Spines in 1211 Asymptomatic (no pain) Subjects

Lumbar Spine
Imaging findings of spine degeneration are present in high proportions of asymptomatic individuals, increasing with age. Many imaging-based degenerative features are likely part of normal aging and unassociated with pain. These imaging findings must be interpreted in the context of the patient's clinical condition and clinical correlation with the imaging.

A study reporting imaging finding for 3110 asymptomatic individuals found (Brynjikji et al. (2015). Am J Neuroradiology):
- The prevalence of disc degeneration ranged from 37% in asymptomatic individuals in their 20s to 96% of those in their 80s.
- Disc signal loss was present in over 50% of individuals older than 40 years and, by 60 years, 86% of individuals had signal loss of scans.
- Disc height loss and disc bulges increased 1% per year on average.
- Disc protrusions and annular fissures did not substantially increase with age.
- Facet joint degeneration is rare below 40 years of age, and the prevalence increases sharply with ages over 40 years.
- Spondylolisthesis is not commonly found in asymptomatic individuals until 60 years of age, but prevalence doesn't increase greatly until 70-80 years.

Shoulder
Asymptomatic shoulder abnormalities were found in 96% of the subjects. The most common were subacromial-subdeltoid bursal thickening, acromioclavicular joint osteoarthritis, and supraspinatus tendinosis. Ultrasound findings should be interpreted closely with clinical findings to determine the cause of symptoms. Girish et al. (2011). Am J Roent.

Superior labral tears are diagnosed with high frequency using MRI in 45- to 60-year-old individuals with asymptomatic shoulders. These shoulder MRI findings in middle-aged populations emphasize the need for supporting clinical judgment when making treatment decisions for this patient population. To avoid overtreatment, physicians should realize that superior labral tears diagnosed by MRI in individuals between the ages of 45 and 60 years may be normal age-related findings. High Prevalence of Superior Labral Tears Diagnosed by MRI in Middle-Aged Patients with Asymptomatic Shoulders, The Orthopaedic Journal of Sports Medicine, 4(1), January 5, 2016.

Knee

In the study, "Asymptomatic Knees with Osteoarthritis? What to Make of Positive MRI Findings, The British Journal of Sports Medicine, June 9th, 2018. 4,751 participants with a total of 5,397 healthy, non-painful knees were analyzed based on MRI results, healthy, non-painful knees presented with the following odds of having the following osteoarthritic signs:

Chance someone will have any osteoarthritic sign: <40 years old: 4-14% and >40 years old: 19-43%
Chance someone has an articular cartilage defect: 24% overall prevalence
Chance someone has a meniscal tear: 10% overall prevalence
Chance someone has a bone marrow lesion: 18% overall prevalence
Chance someone presents with osteophytes: 25% overall prevalence

The understanding that many findings on MRI are a natural course of aging is important to help educate patients who may want to seek aggressive treatment early following a traffic collision. Care more for the symptoms, rather than basing treatment heavily upon imaging findings. As we get older, it's normal to have some "osteoarthritic changes" that will pop up on MRI, even without pain or symptoms. Although it's true that severe osteoarthritic changes can lead to pain and even arthroplasty, it's important to help educate patients on the possibility of having little to no pain or symptoms with OA despite positive imaging findings, in order to work towards positive change.

MRI CENTERS AND RADIOLOGISTS

Magnetic resonance imaging (MRI) is often perceived as a service where there are no meaningful differences in quality between imaging centers or radiologists, and thus an area in which patients can be advised to select a provider based on price and convenience alone. Based on my experience and a recent study (Variability in diagnostic error rates of 10 MRI centers performing lumbar spine MRI examinations on the same patient within a 3-week period The Spine Journal 17 (2017) 554–561 Herzog, et al), this assumption is not correct, and the assumption that it is can negatively impact patient care, outcomes, and costs.

This study found marked variability in the reported interpretive findings and a high prevalence of interpretive errors in radiologists' reports of an MRI examination of the lumbar spine performed on the same patient at 10 different MRI centers over a short time period. As a result, the authors conclude that where a patient obtains his or her MRI examination and which radiologist interprets the examination may have a direct impact on radiological diagnosis, subsequent choice of treatment, and clinical outcome. Below are some of the findings:

Pathologic Finding	True Positive Rate Sensitivity	False Negative Rate Miss Rate
Anterior spondylolisthesis	90%	10%
Vertebral fracture	70%	30%
Neural foraminal stenosis	67.5%	32.5%
Facet degeneration	62.5%	37.5%
Disc degeneration	60%	40%
Central canal stenosis	55%	45%
Disc herniation	52.5%	47.5%
Nerve root involvement	27.5%	72.5%

A good example of an incidental finding where the radiologist's wording in the report is harmful is the use of the word "tear". Tears can occur, but in most cases, they are fissures rather than tears. Recommendations of the combined task forces of the North American Spine Society, the American Society of Spine Radiology, and the American Society of Neuroradiology state that, "As far back as the 1995 NASS document, authors have recommended that such lesions be termed "fissures" rather than "tears," primarily out of concern that the word "tear" could be misconstrued as implying a traumatic etiology. Because of potential misunderstanding of the term "annular tear," and consequent presumption that the finding of an annular fissure indicates that there has been an injury, the term "annular tear" should be considered nonstandard and "annular fissure" be the preferred term. Imaging observation of an annular fissure does not imply an injury or related symptoms, but simply defines the morphologic change in the annulus.) D.F. Fardon et al. / The Spine Journal 14 (2014) 2525–2545

MALINGERING
Malingering is the intentional production of false or grossly exaggerated physical or psychological symptoms, motivated by external incentives, such as avoiding military duty, avoiding work, obtaining financial compensation, evading prosecution, or obtaining drugs. Pure malingering is the faking of a disease

when it does not exist at all. Partial malingering is the conscious amplification or exaggeration of existing symptoms, or deceitful allegation that prior conditions or symptoms did not exist. Pure malingering and partial malingering are both fraudulent activities. Partial malingering (symptom amplification and avoiding apportionment) is more common and difficult to detect than pure malingering.

The relevance of considering malingering in the clinical assessment of a person with any injuries or complaints arises from the co-occurrence of two necessary factors:
1.   An injury (either physical or psychological) has occurred as a result of a specific event (collision), and
2.   There is an incentive (financial or otherwise) to complain of symptoms.

A fascinating study examined the number of claims for "whiplash" injury in a Canadian province after changing from a system of tort to a no-fault insurance system. The researchers found that the number of whiplash claims fell by almost 30% and the claims were resolved, on average, some 200 days earlier. Longer time to completion was associated with higher initial pain intensity and depression in the claimant but also with non-patient factors, such as engaging the services of a lawyer or seeing health practitioners who were more likely to offer active interventions, perhaps "validating'" the illness perception.

Unlike malingering, somatoform disorders are a medical diagnosis, and the patient is not faking or fraudulent. Somatoform disorders are a group of disorders characterized by symptoms suggesting physical disorders without demonstrable organic findings to explain the symptoms. The symptoms are real and are not under the person's conscious control. Hypochondriacal disorder, somatoform pain disorder, conversion disorder, body dysmorphic disorder, and functional somatic syndromes are examples of somatization disorders. All somatoform disorders co-exist with anxiety and depression.

Conversion disorder is characterized by a symptom(s) suggestive of a neurological disorder that affects sensation or voluntary motor function but is not fully explained by any known general medical condition. The symptom is not consciously or intentionally produced and is severe enough to impair functioning or to require medical attention.

Hypochondriasis is characterized by persistent, health-related worry and magnification of symptoms, despite appropriate medical reassurance and lack of findings on physical or laboratory examination.

Factitious disorders are also relevant in the differential diagnosis. Factitious disorders are a group of disorders characterized by intentional production or feigning of physical or psychological symptoms or signs. The motivation here is related to a need to assume the sick role (e.g. to solicit attention or sympathy), rather than to seek obvious secondary gains, such as economic rewards.

Healthcare providers need to be cognizant to identify malingering and/or somatization and help prevent patients from having unnecessary procedures, prevent fraud, and reduce costs. This is also important to prevent catastrophizing.

DEFINITIONS TO SUPPORT THIS CHAPTER

Symptoms - Any subjective evidence of disease or physiological responses within the body. In contrast, a sign is objective. A departure from normal function or feeling which is noticed by a patient. It should be noted that in most cases pain is a symptom and not a diagnosis.

Signs - is an objective indication of some diagnostic finding or characteristic that may be detected by a patient or anyone (especially a healthcare provider) before, during or after a physical examination of a patient.

History - information gained by a provider by asking specific questions, with the aim of obtaining information useful in formulating a diagnosis and providing care to the patient.

Physical Examination - inspection, palpation, movement, orthopedic testing, neurological testing, strength, and other condition specific procedures.

Subjective - Perceived only by the patient only and not evident to the examiner.

Objective - observable and measurable data ("signs") obtained through observation, physical examination, laboratory and diagnostic testing.

Pathology - The study of disease.

Pathognomonic - means characteristic for a particular disease. A pathognomonic sign is a particular sign whose presence means that a particular disease is present beyond any doubt.

Diagnosis - is the process of determining which disease or condition explains a person's signs and symptoms. A diagnosis is based on information from sources such as findings from a physical examination, consultation, medical history, clinical findings, diagnostic tests and clinical reasoning.

Differential diagnosis - A list of possible diagnoses from most likely to least likely. It is used to guide further assessments, testing and possible treatment.

Working diagnosis - The highest diagnosis on the list of the differential diagnosis, the most probable diagnosis.

Clinical correlation - The signs, symptoms, exam findings, orthopedic testing and diagnostic testing are in agreement with the most logical diagnosis.

Patient selection - the findings, diagnosis, treatment and the patient are suitable for a successful outcome.

Pain generator - The primary anatomical or physiological cause of pain.

Tissue damage pain - Tissue injury with inflammation results in the release of various mediators that cause pain. Also referred to as acute pain, nociceptive pain, warning pain or Eudynia.

Acute-on-chronic pain - acute condition superimposed on an underlying chronic condition.

Aggravation - A permanent worsening of a prior condition.

Exacerbation - A temporary worsening of a prior condition. The condition is expected to return to a baseline.

Precipitation - Accident caused a new injury or condition for which the claimant was at risk, but may have never developed.

Acceleration - Speeds the course of the disease, which would have become symptomatic, was more rapid due to injury. Disease not worse than it would be without the trauma just occurs sooner.

Recurrence - Reappearance of signs and symptoms attributed to a prior condition.

Primary pain generator - The tissue or anatomical structure damaged by disease or trauma. Examples of pain generators are joints affected by bones, joints, muscles, cancer, skin damaged by a burn or organs. Once the specific pain generator is identified the condition can be treated in a more specific manner. If back pain is being caused by a kidney stone but treatment is being rendered for a disc pathology, the primary pathology will still cause pain.

Idiopathic - of unknown cause.

Nociceptive pain - pain that is invoked by noxious stimulation of structures and tissue.

Psychogenic pain - physical pain that is caused, increased, or prolonged by mental, emotional, or behavioral factors.

Nonorganic - Nonorganic is a term used to describe an apparently physical disorder that in fact is not arising from the organ or body part but from an abnormality of the use or presentation of that body part.

Neurogenic pain - pain due to dysfunction of the peripheral or central nervous system, in the absence of nociceptor stimulation by trauma or disease.

Viscerogenic pain - Damage, pathology or trauma of visceral origin can be referred to the corresponding somatic areas. Cardiac pain is a good example. Cardiac pain is not felt in the heart but is referred to areas supplied by the corresponding spinal nerves.

Myofascial pain - pain in muscles or fascia (a type of connective tissue that surrounds muscles). It can occur in distinct, isolated areas of the body. Because any muscle or fascia in the body may be affected, this may cause a variety of localized symptoms.

Dermatomal or Radicular pain - A dermatome is an area of skin supplied by sensory neurons that arise from a spinal nerve ganglion. Symptoms that follow a dermatome (e.g. like pain or a rash) may indicate a pathology that involves the related nerve root. Radicular pain is distinctive, having a lancinating quality and traveling along the length of the limb in a band no wider than two or three inches. This is the only pain that has been produced by stimulating nerve roots. Radiculopathy often presents with a non-standard patterns.

Sclerotome or Somatic pain - Pain from somatic tissues. Somatic referred pain is perceived in regions innervated by nerves other than those that innervate the site of noxious stimulation – the core of the definition of referred pain. It is produced by noxious stimulation of nerve endings within spinal structures such as discs, facet joints, or sacroiliac joints. The mechanism does not involve nerve roots; it involves convergence on second-order neurons in the spinal cord. As a general rule, somatic referred pain is perceived in regions that share the same segmental innervation as the source.

Neuroplastic pain (Maldynia) - Classified as a form of neuropathic pain, chronic pain or maldynia. Refers to pain caused by or pain increased because of changes within the nervous system. These structural and functional changes can occur at every level of the nervous system.

Malingering - The fabrication of symptoms of mental or physical disorders for a variety of reasons, such as: financial compensation (often tied to fraud); avoiding school, work, or military service; or obtaining drugs. Failure to detect actual cases of malingering imposes an economic burden on health care systems and insurance carriers.

Factitious disorder - a pattern of behavior centered on the exaggeration or outright falsifications of one's own health problems, or the health problems of others. Some people with this disorder fake or exaggerate physical problems; others fake or exaggerate psychological problems, or a combination of physical and psychological problems. Factitious disorder differs from malingering. While malingerers make their claims out of a motivation for personal gain, people with factitious disorder have no such motivation.

Somatoform disorder - Involves persistent complaints of varied physical symptoms that have no identifiable physical origin. The person is not "faking." Somatization disorder is a medical problem. The disorder, however, is probably related to brain function or emotional regulation rather than the area of the body that has become the focus of the patient's attention. The symptoms are real and are not under the person's conscious control.

FURTHER READING TO SUPPORT THIS CHAPTER

Bates' Guide to Physical Examination and History Taking 12th edition.

ODG Guidelines from Work Loss Data Institute, 2018

Weiner's Pain Management: A Practical Guide for Clinicians, 6th edition. Mark V. Boswell, B. Eliot Cole

Whiplash and Mild Traumatic Brain Injury, Arthur C. Croft , Spine Research Institute of Sa; 1st edition (2009)

Whiplash-Associated Diseases, American Medical Association, , Rene Cailliet, 2007

Motor Vehicle Collision Injuries, Second Ed, Lawrence Nordhoff, Jones & Bartlett Publishers 2005

"The Anatomy & Biomechanics of Acute and Chronic Whiplash Injury", Traffic Injury Prevention, 10: 2, 101-112

Whiplash: evidence base for clinical practice, Michele Sterling PhD, Churchill Livingstone, 2011

American Medical Association: Disability Evaluation, second edition. Chicago, AMA 2003.

American Medical Association: Guides to the Evaluation of Permanent Impairment, sixth edition. Chicago, American Medical Association, Mosby, 2007. (Also fifth edition published in 2000)

Photographic Manual of Regional Orthopaedic and Neurologic Tests by Joseph J. Cipriano DC

Differential Diagnosis and Management for the Chiropractor 5th Edition, by Thomas A. Souza DC

Netter's Orthopaedic Clinical Examination: An Evidence-Based Approach (Netter Clinical Science) 3rd Edition, by Joshua Cleland

Joint Structure and Function: A Comprehensive Analysis Fifth Edition by Pamela K. Levangie DPT, Cynthia C. Norkin DPT

CHAPTER 5
PREVENTING CHRONIC PAIN FOLLOWING TRAFFIC COLLISIONS

Anticipating pain is worse than feeling it.
Chronic pain is more than a hurt; it is to all too many a way of life.
If you think that you will get better, you are halfway to recovery.
With proper management, many patients can fully recover from their injuries.
Catastrophizing, fear, & worry about pain will actually create the very pain that you fear.

SUMMARY – This chapter is specially designed to prevent acute pain from turning into chronic pain after traffic collisions. This information is the result of treating over 8,000 acute and chronic pain patients over the past 20 years. These recommendations are also consistent with the current science of acute and chronic pain. First, let's recap (because repetition is the mother of all learning) acute and chronic pain.

Acute pain is generally defined as being caused by an identifiable source that is typically associated with some degree of tissue damage, inflammation, or disease process. Acute pain has a relatively brief duration, usually a few days or weeks, and most often serves a warning of tissue damage. Acute tissue damage typically heals in a predictable timeframe for each tissue type. Severe structural pathology from any permanent impairments or potentially life-threatening conditions needs to be identified.

Chronic pain is defined as pain that lasts beyond the expected period of tissue healing. It is often described as pain lasting longer than 3 months, but this time period is a rule of thumb; typical healing time for each tissue type and individual variances should be considered. Since the tissue that was damaged has healed, chronic pain is best understood as a separate disease from acute pain. Preventing acute pain from turning into chronic pain is essential to solving the pain epidemic.

There is often a disconnect between impairment and disability. Some patients with severe tissue damage and ratable impairment have very little long-term pain or disability, while some patients with little or no tissue damage develops chronic pain and disability. Why? This chapter will help to explain the disconnect and help the suffering patient heal.

Please understand that pain is not just about the tissue damage. There are many incidental findings or pathologies that do not produce pain or dysfunction. Invasive procedures intended to "fix" incidental pathologies, that are not the pain generator, are dangerous and harmful. A key conceptual shift is that chronic pain is the end result. Pain is an output of the brain, designed to protect you, like an alarm system. In fact, chronic pain is like an alarm system that won't shut off.

This is important because "conventional" treatment or management of chronic conditions including pain has been a failure and the problem is getting worse. (Just look at our opioid epidemic) One of the greatest obstacles to pain relief is that most of our beliefs about what causes chronic pain are in fact erroneous. For successful treatment of chronic pain there are 5 major realizations:
1. Acute and chronic pain are (in most cases) different pathologies with different mechanisms.
2. Structural pathologies are often not the true cause of the chronic pain following traffic collisions.
3. Proper management of acute injuries and pain can prevent chronic pain development.
4. Conventional treatment of chronic pain is not working and has been a failure.
5. Successful treatment of chronic pain must include significant patient involvement.

Pain is often "overprotective." Reassurance that the danger implied by pain may be overstated is a path to break the chains of chronic pain. Letting the pain go and not attaching to pain is essential. Attachment to the pain, stress, and negative self-talk leads to suffering. Focus on flourishing in health and happiness, not the pain. Let the pain and events that caused the acute pain go. Do what is needed for healing of any tissue damage.

Acute tissue damage pain from traffic collisions is common and typically heals within 6-12 weeks of the injury. Severe tissue damage that would be considered permanent impairment is the exception. The sooner you or the patient reduce pain or symptoms, normalize motion, and return to normal health, the less likely the acute pain is to advance into chronic pain. The 4 recommendations below (the secret sauce) should be used as first line treatment for acute traffic injuries:
1. Reassure - Rule out serious tissue damage and reassure that there is no permanent pathology. Reduce fear and anxiety.
2. Reduce pain and inflammation- Acute pain relief, reduce inflammation, and promote tissue healing.
3. Stay active - Get back to usual activities, move, and work.

4. Promote health – Normalize range of motion, strengthen, eat a healthy diet, drink only water, sleep, and be mindful.

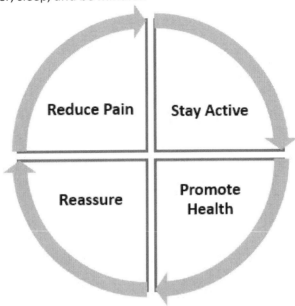

When applicable, "one of the most important things that a doctor can say to a patient is that you are going to be fine." One of the worst things that a doctor or healthcare provider can do is to fuel the fire of catastrophizing. Invasive procedures such as surgery are rarely needed following a traffic collision. If the tissue damage is not life-threatening then stay calm and don't worry about the pain but do whatever is necessary to heal or fix the injured tissue. The goals are to promote tissue healing, reduce pain, normalize range of motion, and strengthen.

The things that we do, the way that we think, and the way we behave will have an important role in our health and recovery. Whether you want to believe it or not, you are in control of your health and you must take an active role. "We are all in control of our individual health, but only the healthy will admit it." If you are sick and tired of being sick and tired, then take control and get healthy. Taking responsibility for your personal health and happiness is not just your duty, but it's your obligation!

In many traffic injuries, the patient may have preexisting pain or pathology that can complicate healing. The same recommendations should be followed for acute tissue damage pain with additional protocols for chronic pain relief. In most cases, focusing on creating happiness and health versus stopping the pain is very productive.

INTRODUCTION

It's well established that the risk factors for acute injury or pain are often different than the risk factors for chronic pain following traffic collisions. Preventing acute pain's transformation to chronic pain is essential to combating our chronic pain epidemic. As the saying goes, "an ounce of prevention is worth a pound of cure".

Neck pain, back pain, headaches, and other musculoskeletal symptoms are a leading cause of disability in the US and worldwide. In traffic collisions approximately 50% of occupants walk away with slight to no pain and do not seek treatment. Studies show that of the 50% of occupants that seek treatment or have more significant acute pain, approximately 25-50% of these people progress to chronic pain or long-term symptoms. Remember that chronic symptoms are defined as symptoms beyond typically 3 months. Approximately 2-5% of the injured occupants are left with permanent impairments.

Interestingly, patients who have no pain (asymptomatic) at 3 months continue to have no pain (attributed to the collision) at 2 year follow ups. This is why we work hard to get patients pain-free and moving well as soon as possible.

One of my favorite mantras is, "A good diagnosis is the first step to a great treatment". Diagnosis of the anatomical & structural tissue damage is essential for proper patient management and better for better outcomes. Structural pathologies such as impairment, severe tissue damage, deconditioning, tissue tensile strengthen, past surgeries, stenosis, arthritis, weakness, atrophy, and more all can contribute to chronic pain. I have seen many cases where chronic pain exists because the provider was awful at diagnosing what's wrong with the patient or managed the patient's care improperly.

Chronic inflammation, psychological factors, healthcare choices, and lack of general health are also driving forces behind chronic pain and should be addressed early in care. It is often more important to know what sort of person a disease has, than to know what sort of a disease a person has. It's not a coincidence that the same risk factors for diabetes, heart disease, stroke, cancer, and other chronic diseases are also common in chronic pain patients. Sedentary lifestyle, sitting too long, obesity, poor eating habits, lack of sleep, and mental dysfunctions are major causes of disease.

There are many pathways and theories concerning chronic pain and disease, but this chapter will go over the most commonly accepted. The first part of this chapter will discuss the main causes of chronic pain, then we will discuss strategies to prevent chronic pain, and finally what to do if chronic pain progresses.

PAIN EXPERIENCE

Pain is not just a message from injured tissues but a complex experience that is thoroughly tuned by your brain. The perception of pain is an extremely individual and unique aversive experience associated with actual or potential tissue damage with sensory, emotional, cognitive, and social components. Clinically, pain is whatever the patient says he or she is experiencing whenever he or she says it occurs.

Remember from the chapter on pain that there are two different pathways in our brains that contribute to the pain experience:
The first pain pathway sends signals through nerves about the intensity of painful stimuli to a number of regions in the brain that have typically been associated with pain perception, such as the anterior cingulate cortex. This pathway is how we typically think about acute pain and tissue damage.

The second pathway mediates the effects of mind (cognitive) regulation on pain perception and involves increasing activity in the medial prefrontal cortex and nucleus accumbens. These are brain regions are associated with emotion, motivation, neuroplastic changes, and perceptions of pain in the body. This second pathway holds some of the keys to understanding the "psychosocial " aspects of debilitating pain or suffering.

Research shows that predictive coding and how our nervous system is "wired" actually predicts or expects pain following traffic collisions. According to the predictive coding model, the brain is always building and refining its mental maps of the outside world and our bodies. Our perceptions depend in large part on these mental maps, not just incoming sensory data. The predictive coding framework helps explain why pain is affected by past experiences, advertising, thoughts, expectations, and emotions, and not just tissue damage. The way that you are wired (your nervous system) and software (your mind) may be prewired or preprogrammed for pain and particularly pain following traffic collisions.

In many cases the tissue injury by itself is not enough to explain the reported ongoing pain and disability. This can often result in conflict concerning an injury claim and possibly unnecessary procedures if the provider is not in tune with the cause of the pain. The pain has to do with the tissue damage combined with the state of the brain and the nervous system. The more emotionally and cognitively the brain reacts to the initial injury, the more likely the pain will persist after the injury has healed. If the tissue damage is not life-threatening, then don't worry about the pain but do whatever is necessary to heal the injured tissue.

Pain x (Catastrophizing + Attachment + Resistance) = Suffering. Catastrophizing about the pain, attaching to the pain, and resisting the realty of your life creates suffering and more pain. Things can get blown out of proportion very quickly. This has also been described by Eckhart Tolle as the pain-body. The pain-body is an accumulation of stress, negativity, fear, and old emotional wounds that affect our health and sense of well-being; physically, emotionally, mentally, and energetically. It's a state of consciousness that is self-destructive and addicted to unhappiness.

The primary cause of the suffering and unhappiness is never the situation but your thoughts and interpretations of it. This causes an arising of the ego. The ego is a psychological construct, it's a story, it's a false self, it's an image created in the mind which is deluded into looking at itself as a "separate" entity. The ego can also be defined simply as a dysfunctional relationship with the present moment. In this state of mind, you are no longer in control, but spotting the ego is the first step to getting control back.

It's important to recognize that the perception or expectation of pain is often greater than the actual tissue damage. It is very clear the mind alters pain perceptions, and it's exciting that the experience of pain involves multiple brain pathways and can be self-regulated. Pain catastrophizing, expectations, predictive coding, beliefs, and behaviors have been found to be related to ongoing pain and disability. Catastrophizing, fear, and worry about pain will actually create the very pain crisis that you fear.

The intensity of initial complaints is one identifiable factor related to the severity and persistence of ongoing pain. Some common emotional responses to pain can include anxiety, depression, anger, feeling misunderstood, and demoralization. Significant tissue damage and the quality of healthcare all play a role in the management of traffic injury pain. Below are some of the possible variables associated with traffic injuries and progression to chronic pain:

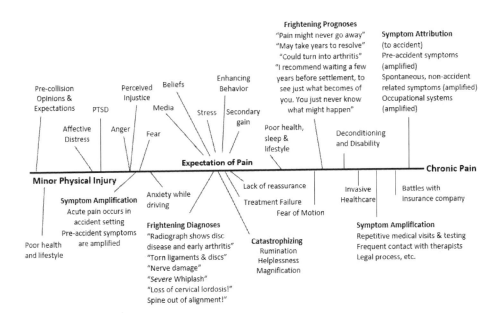

Great examples of the powerful effect of psychological processes on pain are the placebo and nocebo effects. Placebo and nocebo effects are presumably psychogenic, but they can induce measurable changes in the body and the brain. Expectation and previous experience are key mediators of placebo or nocebo effects. **Avoid a nocebo effect and promote a placebo effect.**

The placebo and nocebo responses are the result of a complex set of sociocultural beliefs, expectations, and conditioning behaviors, which influence the brain and nervous system. Science has proven that it's possible to induce alterations of pain perception by a purely psychological placebo and nocebo effects. Advertising promoting pain and compensation following traffic collisions is one example that can result in the nocebo effect. The placebo effect is very established in the medical literature and public perception; however, the nocebo effects are equally important.

A nocebo is a negative expectation for a treatment, diagnosis, or prognosis following a traffic collision. For example, an expectation of pain may induce anxiety, which in turn causes the release of cholecystokinin, which facilitates pain transmission. Nocebo effects are defined as adverse events related to negative expectations and learning processes that are involved in the modulation of the brain and descending pain pathways. Research over the last couple of decades has illustrated that behavioral, psycho-neurobiological, and functional changes occur during nocebo-induced pain processing. Nocebo can also be induced by providers or early diagnostic testing that may show incidental pathology. The nocebo effect is a gateway to catastrophizing.

A few years ago, researchers did an experiment with 51 volunteers who were involved in a fake rear-end collision (virtually no forces were transferred to the occupant). 19.6% of the occupants reported "whiplash-like" symptoms 3 days after the sham collision and 9.8% reported pain 4 weeks post "collision". The nocebo effect is a likely explanation of the reported symptoms since the forces involved were not significant enough to cause tissue damage.

A placebo is a positive expectation that may produce a beneficial, healthful, pleasant, or desirable effect. Educating the public that most occupants in traffic collisions are not severely hurt or get better within a few weeks would be extremely helpful in reducing pain following traffic collisions. Providers reassuring patients that the tissue damage will heal could involve corresponding changes in the prefrontal cortex and limbic system, which then produce a cascade of psychophysiological responses, that lead to having no pain or a reduction of pain.

A traffic collision can be a frightening and sometimes even terrifying experience. Therefore, it's not surprising that such an experience often gives rise to post-traumatic anxiety symptoms. Experiencing a traumatic event can also lead to the onset of a so-called acute stress disorder (ASD). The essential features of ASD are the development of anxiety as well as dissociative and other symptoms that occur within one month after exposure to an extreme traumatic stressor.

Following the American Psychiatric Association's DSM IV classification, the specific diagnosis requires several criteria, including derealization, depersonalization, or dissociative amnesia, where an important aspect of the trauma cannot be recalled; recurrent images, thoughts, dreams, illusions, or flashback episodes; and marked avoidance of stimuli that arouse recollections of the trauma. Also, when the formal diagnostic criteria are not met, there can obviously still be acute stress symptoms.

Stress symptoms that persist for more than one month may eventually evolve into a post-traumatic stress disorder (PTSD). PTSD is an anxiety disorder that requires a response of fear at the time of trauma together with three symptom clusters: re-experiencing, avoidance, and hyperarousal symptoms. Mild PTSD is a relatively common condition following traffic collisions.

Consciously or subconsciously, there is also a financial incentive for reporting continued pain and disability following traffic collisions. If symptom amplification or magnification is present, it's the provider's duty to identify this and reassure the patient that there is no serious pathology. A review of the past history, current history, reported symptoms, exam findings, and clinical correlation with diagnostic testing is essential to help determine causation related to the reported collision. There may be incidental findings or pathologies that do not produce pain or dysfunction. Invasive procedures intended to "fix" incidental pathologies that are not the pain generator can make things worse.

HOW LONG DOES IT TAKE TISSUE DAMAGE / ACUTE PAIN TO HEAL

A common question is, "How long does it take for an injury take to heal?" My answer is always the same. It depends on:

1. The type of tissue injured (muscle, ligament, bone, nerve, etc.). Each tissue type has a general range that it takes to heal.
2. Severity of tissue damage or grade of injury. What needs to be done to fix the structural damage?
3. Patient factors that can delay or complicate healing such as; lupus, RA, OA, diabetes, and many other factors.
4. Acute-on-chronic conditions or relapses can also take longer to heal.

For example, a minor cut on the finger might take 4 days to heal in a healthy individual or 12 days in an individual with poor healing. A simple cervical strain in a healthy individual can take 4-8 weeks to heal. A severe broken bone takes up to 2-6 months to heal and up to a year to fully remodel. Trauma that results in more severe tissue damage or permanent impairment also can result from traffic collisions and should be treated appropriately.

Most tissue damage caused by traffic collisions heals within 12 weeks. This would fall within the acute and subacute periods. Continued pain past 12 weeks should have an anatomical cause, with more extensive tissue damage or factors that would explain the delay in healing. Remember that chronic pain is pain that persists beyond the expected time for healing.

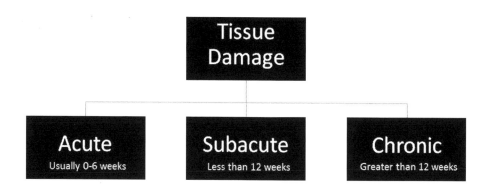

The healing of damaged tissue is a complex and dynamic process, consisting of four primary phases: blood clotting (hemostasis), inflammation, tissue growth (proliferation), and tissue remodeling (maturation). Typically, most tissues heal within 3 months, but some tissue can take up to a year to regain full tensile strength. Recovery from tissue damage includes the resolution of healing (particularly inflammation) and attenuation of nociceptive excitation.

It's also important to remember that more than one tissue type can be injured at the same time. The human body has the power to heal itself from the cellular level up. Pain or symptoms past 3-4 months typically would have tissue damage more severe, such as a permanent impairment. Below is a chart with general estimates (not absolute) of healing times for some common traffic injuries:

Typical Healing Times		
General Muscle Soreness 0 – 3 days Minor Cuts 7 – 14 days Minor Contusions 7 – 14 days Headaches 2-12 weeks Bursitis 2-12 weeks	Tendonitis Nerve Irritation Facet Injury (with no capsular tears) Dislocations PTSD weeks+	2-12 weeks 4-12 weeks 4-12 weeks 4-12 weeks 4-16
Muscle Strain	Grade 1: Grade 2: Grade 3:	0 – 2 weeks 4 days – 12 weeks 6 weeks – 6 months
Ligament Sprain	Grade 1: Grade 2: Grade 3:	0 – 7 days 4 weeks – 12 weeks 6 weeks – 6 months
Bone Injury 6 weeks – 3 months	Disc Injury	6 weeks – 6 months
Concussion 6 weeks – 6 months	Nerve Injury	6 weeks – 6 months
Permanent Impairment / Permanent Damage **4 months+ of pain or symptoms** Any condition that requires surgery, objective evidence of permanent tissue damage or a permanent impairment based on the American Medical Association: Guides to the Evaluation of Permanent Impairment, sixth edition (AMA GUIDES®).		

Severe nerve, brain, bone, visceral, or vascular pathology are rare, but if present, require immediate attention. Early imaging is likely to be of little use in the vast majority of traffic injury cases; with the natural course, most people will recover with conservative measures. There is an assortment of anatomical and psychosocial factors leading to chronic pain, but conceptually there are 2 basic categories of chronic pain:

1. Chronic pain due to a clinically identifiable pain generator.
This type of chronic pain is due to a clearly identifiable cause. Certain structural spine conditions (for example, fracture, cancer, degenerative disc disease, spinal stenosis, ligament instability, and spondylolisthesis) can cause ongoing pain

until successfully treated. These conditions are due to a diagnosable anatomical problem with clinical correlation. In these cases, invasive procedures such as extensive therapy, injections, or surgery may be needed. Over time, a cascade of changes can by initiated by tissue damage which elicits a collection of synaptic, neurotransmitter, and modulatory events that mimics synaptic plasticity and remodeling similar to that seen in learning and memory.

Flareups, exacerbations, and reinjury also fall into this category following collisions. There are many incidental findings or pathologies that do not produce pain or dysfunction. Invasive procedures intended to "fix" incidental pathologies that are not clinically the pain generator are dangerous and harmful.

2. Chronic pain with no significant identifiable pain generator.
This type of pain continues beyond the point of tissue healing and there is no clearly identifiable pain generator that explains the pain. It is often termed "chronic benign pain." Pain can set up a pathway in the nervous system and this becomes the problem in and of itself. The dysfunction in the nervous system sends a pain signal even though there is no ongoing tissue damage.

A COMMON CAUSE OF CHRONIC PAIN SYNDROME AFTER TRAFFIC INJURY
The experience of pain is shaped by a host of different factors such as the extent of tissue damage, area of tissue damage, psychological factors, expectations, catastrophizing, and more. Our response to the stimulus of pain is a major factor between a successful recovery and chronic pain. Of course, any tissue damage that results in a permanent impairment has a higher risk of developing chronic symptoms.

Acute pain commonly occurs following traffic collisions where tissue damage is sustained, such as a broken arm or sprained neck. This pain is helpful because it warns the body of tissue or structural damage. Significant tissue damage that would be considered a potential permanent impairment under the AMA GUIDES® must be screened for. In some cases, structural pathology such as capsular ligament tears can progress to degeneration and arthritic pain. Tissue damage absolutely has a factor in pain and needs to be properly evaluated. The treating provider also has to be aware and not enable opportunistic claimants only out for financial gain.

Again, chronic pain persists beyond the expected time and indicated point of tissue healing and is typically defined as longer than 3 months duration. While pain is present and may feel identical to acute pain, the experience does not have the same meaning. One framework of chronic pain and the pain experience is an integrated relationship between neurological factors, biological factors, sociocultural, and psychosocial cultural factors. The brain and nervous system learns and expects pain because of neuroplasticity.

The three main constructs of chronic pain are: (1) neurological factors such as neuroplastic changes, trauma, inflammation, chemical factors, and certain diseases; (2) biological factors such as genetic / epigenetics, tissue damage, structural pathology, impairment, inflammation, chemical factors, and certain diseases; and (3) psychosocial and cultural factors such as anxiety, PTSD, depression, catastrophizing, coping strategies, behaviors, social learning, expectations, cognitive bias, predictive coding, family history, perceived injustice, and cultural factors. Please remember that there are some things that we don't even know that we don't know cause disease and pain. Below is my cogwheel of chronic pain which is a simplistic depiction of many, but by no means all, the factors associated with chronic pain.

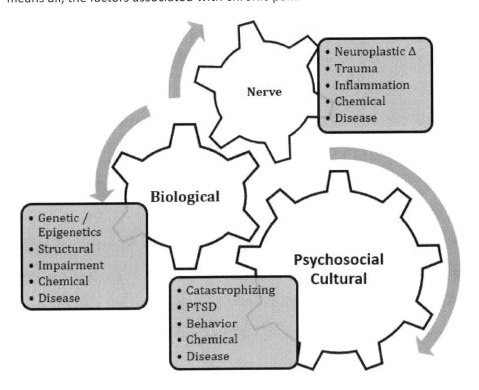

Neurological Factors
Certain diseases, trauma, tissue damage, chemical imbalances, and neuroplastic changes (occurring at any level of the nervous system) can cause pain or magnify pain. Chronic inflammation and chemical irritation is also a common

driving force behind acute and chronic pain. Getting this inflammation under control is a good starting point for dealing with pain.

Neuroplastic changes in structure and function are not only a consequence of chronic pain but are involved in the preservation of pain. Your pain warning system is not just a system for the conduction of pain impulses from the periphery to the brain. Scientists now know that changes can take place in the receptors, nerves, spinal cord, and higher brain centers following tissue damage. Inflammation, continued use of the pain system, disuse of inhibiting factors, and learned behaviors all can lead to chronic pain. The way that your nervous system is wired and the way your mind is programmed has an influence on your pain.

Research has also shown that your brain learns to predict or expect pain. Brain imaging (for example, functional MRI, PET, EEG and magnetoencephalography) is widely considered to have potential for diagnosis, prognostication, and prediction of treatment outcome in patients with chronic pain. "Our brain is the most powerful tool that we have in medicine; the only problem is that we lost the instruction manual" (until now).

Biological Factors
There is credible evidence from twin and population-based studies that genetic risk factors can explain some of the individual differences in pain perception and the etiology of chronic pain conditions. Epigenetics is the study of biological mechanisms that will switch genes on and off. Epigenetic mechanisms enhance or suppress gene expression without alterations of the primary DNA sequence. Epigenetic mechanisms have been shown to be involved in synaptic plasticity, learning, and memory, as well as depression, fear, anxiety, and catastrophizing. The spinal cord and brain can undergo injury-induced changes in gene expression that are mediated by epigenetic mechanisms and potentially contribute to pain syndromes. Thus, epigenetic mechanisms present dynamic processes for controlling changes in neuronal activity and behavior that may be responsible for the persistent manifestation of a chronic pain state.

Epigenetics research is very promising and will be a mainstay in disease prevention for years to come. What you eat, where you live, who you interact with, when you sleep, how you think, how you exercise, and even aging – all can cause chemical modifications around the genes that will turn those genes on or off over time. The good news is that you have more control over your genes than previously thought.

Putting toxins and poisons into our body is a frequent cause of symptoms. The things that we put in our body, including the foods that we eat (particularly sugar), cause chronic inflammation in the body resulting in pain. Sugar is toxic and is a major contributor to obesity, diabetes, heart disease, epigenetics changes, and chronic pain. Chronic inflammation is commonly attributed to eating CRAP: C – Carbonated Drinks; R – Refined Sugar; A – Artificial Sweeteners, Artificial Colors, and Alcohol; and P – Processed Foods. Smoking triggers an immunologic response to vascular injury, which is associated with chronic inflammation and pain.

Structural pathologies such as impairment, severe tissue damage, deconditioning, tissue tensile strength, past surgeries, stenosis, arthritis, weakness, atrophy, and more all can contribute to chronic pain. Chemical, endocrine, and inflammatory dysfunctions also play a role in chronic pain. Of course, diseases such as arthritis, RA, OA, lupus, diabetes, disc herniations, facet capsular tears, and more can delay healing. Any condition with severe tissue damage that would qualify for a permanent impairment rating by the AMA GUIDES® can contribute to chronic pain or symptoms.

Psychosocial Cultural Factors
In the past 20 years, psychosocial factors have shown to be a major feature of chronic pain following traffic injuries. These factors include: anxiety, PTSD, TBI, distress, depression, catastrophizing, coping strategies, behaviors, social learning, expectations, cognitive bias, predictive coding, family history, perceived injustice, and cultural factors. As pain becomes chronic, the sensory components become less important and the emotional and behavioral components tend to take on more importance.

Post-traumatic stress disorder (PTSD) is a mental health condition that occurs in at least 15-20% of motor vehicle collision survivors who have sustained a physical injury. PTSD and panic disorder are often intertwined and concurrent with chronic pain. Post-traumatic stress disorder is a diagnosis given to distressed individuals who have been exposed to some event that threatens their life or physical well-being. Clinically, it is essential to differentiate between post-traumatic stress disorder (PTSD), mild traumatic brain injury (TBI), and chronic pain syndrome (CPS). These conditions can lead to long-term symptoms if not properly managed.

There is a negative stigma to saying that the pain is "all in your head," but by definition, all pain is in your head. Psychological factors such as perceptions (catastrophizing), emotions (depression), and pain-related behaviors (avoidance) can influence perceived pain intensity, physical function, and treatment outcomes. Below is an example of a psychosocial and cultural model for recovery after a typical injury. One path leads to a recovery and the other into the chronic pain cycle.

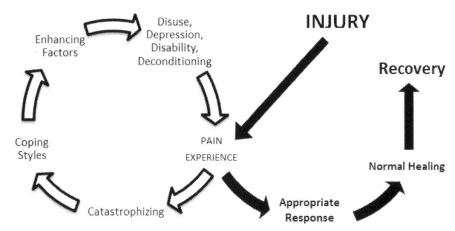

Pain Experience

After the injury or tissue damage the first "fork in the road" is the pain experience. As discussed earlier, the pain experience can be positive and appropriate for the extent of tissue damage or negative, leading to catastrophizing. As a provider this is the most important time to get the patient on the right track psychologically. A patient who attaches to the pain, negatively judges the pain, catastrophizes, or focuses on the pain gets more pain. Remember, Pain x (Catastrophizing + Attachment + Resistance) = Suffering.

Doctors are a guide in helping the patient recover physically and emotionally. Providers that are not in tune with this can push the patient to catastrophizing by early testing, fear, invasive procedures, unnecessary surgery, and lack of reassurance. Providers reassuring patients that the tissue damage will heal could involve corresponding changes in the prefrontal cortex and limbic system, which then produce a cascade of psychophysiological responses that lead to having reduced pain or, better yet, no pain. As a provider, sometimes we have to tell patients what they need to know and not what they want to hear.

As seen below; nociception, perception, suffering, and behavior need to be proportional to the tissue damage for an appropriate pain response. Heightened reaction to tissue damage includes: increased perception of pain, suffering, and exaggerated behavior. This is a negative pathway for recovery.

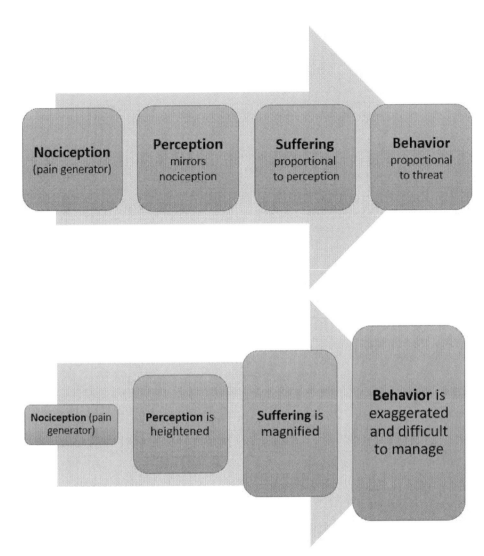

Catastrophizing - Focusing on the pain

Pain catastrophizing is a negative reasoning or belief that the experienced pain will inevitably result in the worst outcome (remember the nocebo effect). A person catastrophizing would expect to have severe pain for the rest of his or her life, even if the tissue damage was mild in severity and was being treated appropriately. Addressing any significant tissue damage by the provider with continual reassurance that the tissue damage will heal is essential to prevent catastrophizing.

Essentially, catastrophizing is making assumptions about what's going on based on very limited or circumstantial evidence. Catastrophizing is characterized by focusing on and magnifying the extent of an actual or anticipated painful stimulus with a negative outlook on recovery. It is a big mistake to make every unwanted aspect of life the symptom of a disorder that needs medication or treatment.

I have found that many patients have ANTs, (automatic negative thoughts). As Henry David Thoreau said, "I have suffered much in my life... and most of it never happened." We create our own suffering by ruminating and magnifying on negative thoughts. Catastrophizing is essentially turning a crisis into a catastrophe. Pain catastrophizing is a multi-dimensional construct comprising magnification, rumination, and helplessness.

Magnification (magnifying the problem) – it can be very easy to blow things out of proportion when you are in intense pain. For example, "this pain is so intense there must be something seriously wrong" or "my spine must be broken". These exaggerated thoughts are often driven by a fear of what might happen in the future, rather than by what is actually happening or likely to happen.

Rumination (over-thinking or obsessing about the problem) - thoughts are dominated by "what if?" and "worst case scenarios." If you focus on the negative aspects of your pain, this increases your feelings of distress. Increased distress leads to increased cortisol & increased pain intensity. Ruminating is simply repetitively going over a thought or obsessing how bad things are. The more we think about, or "ruminate" on, a negative thought, the more entrenched the thought becomes. Negative and traumatic thoughts also tend to "loop." They play themselves over and over until you do something consciously to stop them.

Helplessness (hopeless)– helpless implies having no ability to influence the pain or symptoms or believing there is no positive way to manage. If you ever feel like "I can't go on," or "things will never get better," you probably feel helpless. Feeling helpless not only feels awful, but also can lead you to quit treatment that could help in the long term. Learned helplessness is very common, and the patient does not help themselves.

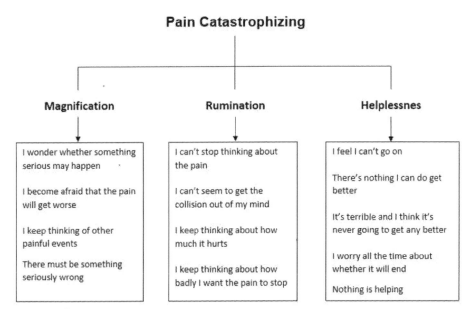

Pain Catastrophizing

Magnification

I wonder whether something serious may happen

I become afraid that the pain will get worse

I keep thinking of other painful events

There must be something seriously wrong

Rumination

I can't stop thinking about the pain

I can't seem to get the collision out of my mind

I keep thinking about how much it hurts

I keep thinking about how badly I want the pain to stop

Helplessnes

I feel I can't go on

There's nothing I can do get better

It's terrible and I think it's never going to get any better

I worry all the time about whether it will end

Nothing is helping

Coping Styles

The catastrophizing response to pain leads into fear-avoidance, passive coping and anger. This results in the experience of heightened pain intensity, increased disability, disuse, depression and difficulty separating from pain.

A common fear-avoidance behavior is kinesiophobia, which refers to the fear of movement. Movement of an injured joint is essential for tissue healing and pain relief. A primary aim of treatment, once the initial trauma has settled, is to regain your full joint, ligament, and muscle range of motion. It is extremely important to dynamically support the muscles surrounding your injury via strengthening exercises. This is important to provide support during the early recovery phase, prevent re-injury, and return you to everyday function. The picture below demonstrates that our mental programing sometimes stops us from doing the things that we need to do to get better.

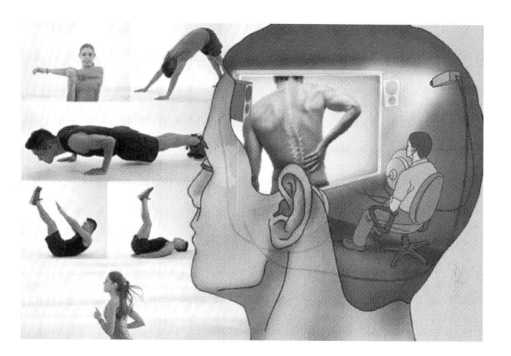

Passive coping includes a low self-efficacy, which is one's belief in one's ability to heal or be pain free. It's a progression of helplessness, and results in dependence on external sources of pain control. These external sources could include medication, therapy, surgeries, street drugs, alcohol, and more. Low self-efficacy can lead people to believe tasks are more difficult than they actually are; they then get discouraged and give up. The helplessness of catastrophizing now progresses to hopelessness.

The ongoing pain, especially with traffic collisions where the occupant was the victim and the pain is due to someone else's negligence, often leads to anger. Some patients remained angry with the person or situation that created the pain. Dealing with the medical legal system and problems caused by the collision add fuel to the fire. Unrelenting anger may create a hypervigilant state of arousal and adds to the magnitude of the pain. In this stage, giving up and pain become a habit.

Possibly one of the most important factors in determining long-term success in addressing chronic pain is achieving a transition from external sources of pain control (medications, providers and a victim mentality) to internal (self) solutions for health and happiness.

Enhancing Factors

Agliophobia is the persistent, unwarranted, and often irrational fear of pain. Fear and anxiety are known to modulate the pain response and cause greater suffering than the physically traumatic stimulus. In this stage, the fear and anxiety of possibly being in pain can often recognize these thoughts as irrational; patients may find it very difficult to keep these thoughts from occurring repeatedly. This kind of phobic thinking can mean that the anxious person inadvertently trains the mind to develop fears of perceived dangers. "I am afraid that I will hurt myself". The fear of pain is often more of a problem than the actual pain experience. This is when the pain becomes suffering.

"I can't stop thinking about how much it hurts!"
"I'm scared the pain will get worse!"
"There's nothing I can do to make it better!"

Focusing on pain and symptoms causes more pain and symptoms. Hypervigilance is an increased state of pain sensitivity accompanied by an increased intensity of behaviors whose purpose is to detect activity. Our thoughts create our world and our words direct our thoughts. Complaining about the pain will neither shorten its duration nor lessen its severity. Hypervigilance may bring about a state of increased anxiety and attention to pain, which can cause pain perception. The research tells us that hypervigilance is a major factor in conditions such as fibromyalgia, chronic low back pain, and irritable bowel syndrome. It tends to start with catastrophic thinking, and results in disuse, depression, disability, and deconditioning.

Disuse, Depression, Disability and Deconditioning
Our thoughts create feelings, our feelings create behavior, and our behavior reinforces thoughts. This process results in disuse, depression, disability, and deconditioning. The fear of motion and fear of pain causes disuse and deconditioning of the body. Hopelessness and depression get worse in this stage as well. All these factors result in significant disability and poor quality of life.

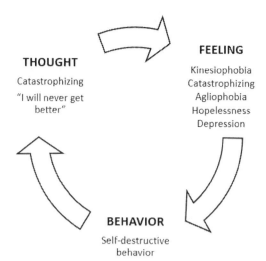

THOUGHT

Catastrophizing

"I will never get better"

FEELING

Kinesiophobia
Catastrophizing
Agliophobia
Hopelessness
Depression

BEHAVIOR

Self-destructive behavior

Depression is due to the difficulties in dealing with pain. It shares many symptoms of major depression including sleep disturbance, fatigue, and cognitive difficulties. Depression connected to the trauma is amplified by catastrophizing, fear, and perceived helplessness behaviors related to pain. This also results in the long-term use of medications, alcohol, and other self-destructive coping mechanisms.

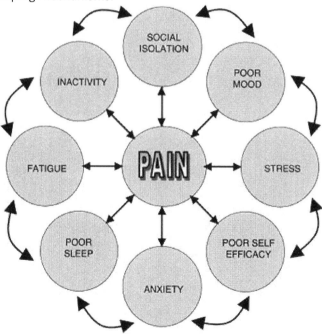

The adage "use it or lose it" is true at all ages. It is a fundamental tenet for health, but even more so following an injury. Deconditioning syndrome is a common but not widely known condition that impacts people after a traumatic injury. The physical and emotional symptoms after an injury due to disuse, disability, inactivity, and immobility lead to deconditioning. Deconditioning not only occurs to the muscles, joints, and ligaments, but also to the cardiovascular system and other body systems. Sedentary lifestyle and sitting too long are major causes of disease.

Complications of Immobility

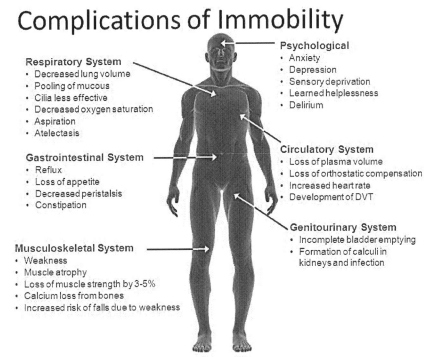

Respiratory System
- Decreased lung volume
- Pooling of mucous
- Cilia less effective
- Decreased oxygen saturation
- Aspiration
- Atelectasis

Gastrointestinal System
- Reflux
- Loss of appetite
- Decreased peristalsis
- Constipation

Musculoskeletal System
- Weakness
- Muscle atrophy
- Loss of muscle strength by 3-5%
- Calcium loss from bones
- Increased risk of falls due to weakness

Psychological
- Anxiety
- Depression
- Sensory deprivation
- Learned helplessness
- Delirium

Circulatory System
- Loss of plasma volume
- Loss of orthostatic compensation
- Increased heart rate
- Development of DVT

Genitourinary System
- Incomplete bladder emptying
- Formation of calculi in kidneys and infection

Inactivity and disuse also leads to weight gain and more musculoskeletal problems. Exercise is one of the best treatments for depression, so lack of exercise fuels depression, anxiety, and fear. As the weeks of inactivity lead into months or years, the negative effects start occurring to the nervous system and cardiovascular system.

You need motion for joint and ligament health. Immobility can lead to joint stiffness, weakness, and an undernourished cartilage, so you need movement to increase blood flow and promote healing. This is why chiropractic works well after an injury. There is a saying in orthopedics that motion is lotion for the joints. If we don't move joints, the synovial fluid (lubrication) for our joints "dries up." What little fluid we do develop isn't absorbed as well by the articular cartilage. This progresses into osteoarthritis!

The deep spinal stabilizing muscles or the deep core are essential for spinal health. The Allcore 360 and daily planks are the best ways to target these muscles. If the body becomes weak and deconditioned, it is more prone to injury and degenerative changes. Deep core weakness and atrophy results in more pain, instability, fear of motion, hypervigilance, catastrophizing, and depression. The cycle of chronic pain continues:

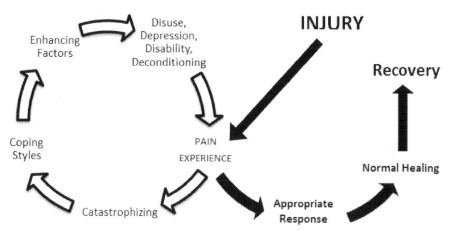

Since we have created a full loop of the chronic pain cycle, it is now time to focus on some solutions to pain including the appropriate pain response. I want you to know that YOU are the most important factor in your health. Take control!

PREVENTING ACUTE PAIN CONVERSION TO CHRONIC PAIN
This is the most important section of this book, because preventing chronic pain is much better than treating chronic pain. Goals are to promote tissue healing, reduce pain, normalize range of motion, and strengthen. Acute tissue damage takes time to heal, but you can take an active role in your recovery by following these five strategies:

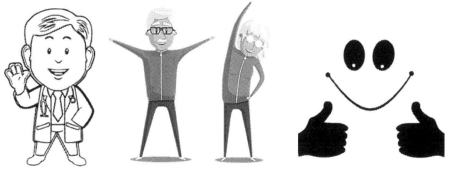

See your Doctor   Stay Active & Keep Moving   Be Positive & Practice Healthy Living

1. If the pain is concerning, see a doctor.
Realize that not all doctors are the same and pick a trusted and experienced doctor. In most cases, x-rays and other tests are not needed for traffic injuries. **Talk to your healthcare provider about what you need to do to recover from your injury.** It is important not to rely solely on medications for complete pain relief. Your medical doctor might recommend that you see a chiropractor, who will treat your condition and give you exercises to help with your recovery. Topical analgesics and short-term therapies are also very effective. Good questions to ask your doctor are:
A. Is anything life-threatening?
B. Is anything broken or does anything require surgery?

If the answer is "no" to these questions, keep calm and focus on healing tissue damage. If a doctor's recommendations do not seem reasonable then get a second opinion. The number one question that you need to ask your doctor is, "would I still need this if this was not a traffic injury case?" Avoid unnecessary early testing such as CT, MRI, or NCV. More than half of requests for MRI of the spine are ordered for indications considered inappropriate or of uncertain value, pointing to evidence of substantial overuse of spine MRI scans. Incidental findings have the potential to frighten patients and initiate cascades of unnecessary surgery or intervention, leading to unnecessary risks.

2. Stay Active.
Do your normal activities to the best of your ability. Although it may be uncomfortable at first, remember that normal activities will not cause any further damage, but will actually speed up your recovery. Remember that some pain and discomfort is normal during the recovery process. You might have to take it easy or do things slower, but stay active. Lying in bed or the couch all day is not going to help. Light duty or wearing a back support for a few days may be helpful. Make sure not to cause more tissue damage.

3. Keep Moving.
Facilitating joint motion after an injury helps with recovery, pain relief, and healing. Ask your chiropractor or physical therapist about the best stretches and exercises for you. After you are able to move the joint with little or no pain, then focus on muscle strengthening. Wearing a neck brace long-term has been shown to cause more harm than good. Motion helps the joint heal and prevents osteoarthritis. It's the golden rule of joint health – the more you move, the less stiffness you'll have.

Noticeable deconditioning or the beginnings of deconditioning start with as little as seven days of complete inactivity. Remember, "use it or lose it". Walking and light exercise is good for the mind and body. The ALLCORE 360 is a great way to dynamically strengthen the deep core spinal stabilizing muscles and so are planks.

4. Be Positive.
A traffic collision can be very stressful and emotional. It's important to stay positive and focus on healing. The vehicle can be fixed or replaced, but you have to live with your body for the rest of your life. Dealing with doctors, insurance companies, and repair shops can be very stressful. Positive thinking is certainly preferable to negative thinking.

Avoid focusing too much on your pain, as it can make your pain more severe. Instead, focus on creating health and happiness. Have an appropriate response for the tissue damage and realistic expectations that healing takes time. Remember that stiffness, aches, and pains are common. Do not allow catastrophizing or fear to lead you into the chronic pain cycle. I have found that truly happy people have the capacity to distract and absorb themselves in activities that divert their energies and attention away from catastrophizing and overthinking symptoms.

5. Practice Healthy Living Habits.
There are certain fundamental basics for good health. Creating healthy habits is essential to recovery. The following are a few tips that will help you heal after an injury:

A. Drink water and only water. Most experts recommend that you drink approximately 80 ounces or more of water a day. This helps the body to heal, gets toxins out of your body, and many other good things.

B. Sleep. Sleep is important for recovery and stress reduction. There isn't one facet of your mental, emotional, or physical performance that's not affected by the quality of your sleep.

C. Stay away from inflammatory foods such as sugar, dairy, caffeine, fast food, gluten, MSG, carbohydrates, vegetable oil, artificial sweeteners, and processed foods. You want to reduce inflammation as much as possible. These foods, principally sugar, will increase inflammation. Chronic inflammation is often a driving force behind chronic pain. Getting this inflammation under control is a good starting point for dealing with pain.

You can also eat foods to reduce inflammation such as: Pineapple, blueberries, avocados, green leafy vegetables, broccoli, celery, beets, salmon, walnuts, coconut oil, flax seeds, turmeric, ginger, chia seeds, almonds, red peppers, black beans, olive oil, tomatoes, spinach, eggs, and garlic.

CHRONIC PAIN TREATMENT STRATEGIES

This section discusses preexisting chronic pain exacerbated by a collision or traffic injuries that have already progressed to chronic pain. Chronic pain and chronic conditions are very difficult to successfully treat, but this section will get you started in the right direction. Disabling and chronic pain can change for the better with some different narratives & coping strategies. Remember that knowledge isn't powerful until it is applied; the purpose of this book is to give you the knowledge to improve your life, but action is fundamental to success. This is your life – make the best of it!

The way that you are wired (your nervous system) and software (your mind) may be prewired or programmed for pain, but the good news is that you can change your wiring and software. Focusing on pain, limitations, and disability will only make problems worse. Of course, you must fix any structural or tissue damage. Flourishing in happiness and health are obtained by changing the things that you do, the way that you think, and your behaviors.

It's difficult to be healthy in an unhealthy society, but the information in this section will give you some of the tools to improve your health and be happy. Additionally, **working with a doctor based on your specific anatomical diagnosis and health conditions is also important.** With chronic conditions, it is critical to know what you can control or fix and what you can't. Do not be disturbed by your diagnosis, but rather by your judgments and opinions about your diagnosis. Many people have arthritis, disc herniations, and other musculoskeletal ailments, nevertheless function normally with little or no pain.

The previous section recommendations for an appropriate response to the tissue damage are also helpful with early treatment of chronic conditions exacerbated by traffic collisions. Promoting tissue healing, reducing pain, normalizing range of motion, and strengthening are all still important. Treatment of chronic conditions relies heavily on patient involvement, and recovery takes much longer than care for acute injury. Related to traffic injuries, the at-fault party is usually responsible for getting you back to pre-accident status, and not necessarily pain-free.

For chronic pain patients focus is less on pain relief and more on principles of successful living. Before we go into some of the steps for obtaining happiness and health, it's important to discuss a few important fundamental principles:

Health
The World Health Organization defines health as a "state of complete physical, mental and social well-being, and not merely the absence of disease or infirmity". This definition has been used by the WHO since 1946 and is still true today. Health also includes the ability to function and adapt to one's environment, injury, or trauma. It has been scientifically proven that what we do, what we eat, and how we act cause health (or can cause disease). Happiness and health are intertwined.

Most patients that I see are, "sick and tired of being sick and tired". Realize that, in most cases, you have more control and influence over your health than any pill, surgery, or injection. Health is our greatest wealth, so please do not squander it.

Happiness
Everyone wants to be "happy," but defining it and being happy is often difficult. Happiness is translated from the Greek concept of eudaimonia, and refers to the good life, good spirit, or flourishing, as opposed to an emotion or feeling that we are accustomed to. Happiness is the result of living every minute with love, grace, gratitude, and purpose.

Happiness comes from within and cannot be traveled to, purchased, owned, earned, worn, or consumed. Happiness is not a goal; it is a by-product of the good life. If you're not happy today, then you won't be happy tomorrow unless you take things into your own hands and take action. You must BE happy before you can BECOME happy. Pursuing "the good life" will help you be healthy and reduce your pain.

Deo Volente
Deo Volente means "God willing," or, "if fate will have it." This is a reserve clause meaning that there are certain things that you cannot control. Approximately 50% of the things that that happen in our lives fall into this category. Accept the things you cannot change and use your power to change the things that you can. Focus on the 50% of your life that you can change rather than the 50% of things that you cannot change.

Flourishing

Flourishing is living within an optimal range of human functioning for an individual. It is a state where people experience positive health, positive emotions, positive psychological functioning, purpose, achievement, and positive social functioning for most of the time. This state represents the fully-functioning individual who is thriving in their life. These individuals realize that they are not perfect, but they are still happy and satisfied with themselves. This contentment does not indicate idleness, however, for these individuals are always striving to achieve their best possible selves.

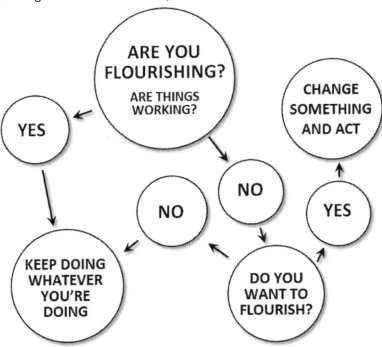

Gratitude
Evidence is mounting that gratitude makes a powerful impact on our bodies, including our immune and cardiovascular health. Higher levels of gratitude are associated with better sleep and with decreased anxiety and depression. According to UCLA's Mindfulness Awareness Research Center, regularly expressing gratitude literally changes the molecular structure of the brain, keeps the gray matter functioning, and makes us healthier and happier. It's physiologically impossible to be in a constant state of gratitude and depressed at the same time.

Action
Action is a fundamental key for success. Knowledge is definitely important, but without action knowledge is powerless. Do not simply be a librarian of

knowledge in the mind but strive to be a warrior of the mind by putting your knowledge into action. Mother Teresa once said, "Praying is prayer plus action." You must either do something that is helpful or stop doing things that are harmful. These are your 2 options: do something or stop doing something. Please remember that time and consistency produce results; many people give up too soon and never see the fruits of their labor.

Action, including inaction, has consequences. Identifying the negative effect of inaction (avoidance of activities, lack of motion, or not getting treatment) or the negative effect of some actions (alcohol, smoking, or reinjury) are important. **A very powerful tool is to list your behaviors, the consequences of your actions or inactions, and then fast forward 5 years to list the outcome of your behaviors.** Investing in your health and happiness will pay you great dividends in 5, 10 and 15 years from now.

Locus of Control
Locus of control is the extent to which you believe that you have power over the events in your lives. A person with an internal locus of control believes that he or she can influence events and their outcomes, while someone with an external locus of control blames others or outside forces which they cannot influence, or believes that chance or fate controls their lives. Examples of external locus are dependency on medications, alcohol, unneeded surgeries, testing, or healthcare providers.

Exercise, good nutrition, sleep, meditation, and a tamed mind are examples of an internal locus. The more that you shift to an internal locus of control, the more control you have over your health and happiness.

Learned Optimism
"Learned optimism" is more than just thinking positive. It's the opposite of "learned helplessness". While he or she might not have control over life's events, what he or she does have control of is his or her own thinking about those events. It's all about the way that you interpret what happens to you. Henry Ford once said, "Whether you think you can or whether you think you can't, you're right." Learning optimism is done by consciously challenging any negative self-talk. I would rather think positive and be wrong some of the time, then be negative and be right all the time!

Maya Angelou went even deeper saying, "if you don't like something, change it. If you can't change it, change your attitude. Don't complain." Accept the things that you cannot change and move on, because when you argue with reality, you lose (but only 100% of the time). Sometimes things happen that may seem negative at the time, but can turn out positive in the long run.

Mindfulness (Being present in the choices that we make)
The mind is the most powerful tool that we have in healthcare. Between stimulus and response, there is a pause. This pause represents our ability to choose a behavior. Being present or mindful in this pause allows us to monitor and alter our thoughts and feelings. Mindfulness starts with embracing the beauty of monotasking. Controlling our thoughts and feelings allows us to dictate our behavior (response). This helps to break the chains of chronic pain.

A positive response or behavior results in flourishing with health and happiness. A negative response leads to pain, suffering, and illness. Below is an example of a positive pathway (mindful) that takes advantage of this pause, giving us power of choice and control over our life and behavior.

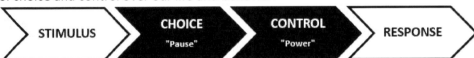

The path below does not take advantage of this pause. The thoughts, feelings, and behavior are on autopilot. We reflexively react to the stimulus and lose control. We forfeit our ability to choose a response, "we do it without thinking". This is an example of a habit, but remember, habits can be helpful or harmful. Take back the control by monitoring your habits and what's going on in your head.

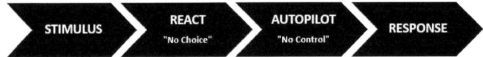

In the pause, listen for negative "self-talk," or our inner voice. Most people don't realize it, but as we go about our daily lives we are constantly thinking about and interpreting the situations we find ourselves in. It's as though we have an internal voice inside our head that determines how we perceive every situation. Psychologists call this inner voice "self-talk," and it includes our conscious thoughts as well as our unconscious assumptions or beliefs. Learning to dispute negative "self-talk" might take time and practice, but is worth the effort.

Once you start looking at your thoughts, you'll probably be surprised by how much of your thinking is inaccurate, exaggerated, or focused on the negatives of the pain or the traffic collision. Habits of thinking need not be forever. One of the most significant findings in psychology in the last thirty years is that individuals can choose the way they think. Guard your mind from faulty or negative programming. Your beliefs, perceptions, and opinions are all influenced by social media, movies, TV, video games, food, music, news, family, friends, and more.

"Name it to tame it" is a powerful mental tool coined by psychiatrist Dr. Daniel Siegel. By putting this simple technique to work, your emotions can inform you and not overwhelm you. Solely naming an emotion moves your thought from the primitive limbic system part of your brain to your prefrontal cortex part of the brain, which is the executive center of the brain. The primitive part of the brain can put you into fight or flight mode, while the more advanced prefrontal cortex gives us the control to make better choices. Labeling your emotion is crucial for decision making and control over behavior.

To reduce pain, we need to reduce the perception of danger and increase perception of safety. This moves control from the reflexive and survival mechanisms of the lower brain to the higher brain. The prefrontal cortex calms pain. Technically speaking, the dorsolateral prefrontal cortex (DLPFC) exerts active control on pain perception by modulating corticosubcortical and corticocortical pathways. But don't worry about the technical process of how this works – just "name it to tame it."

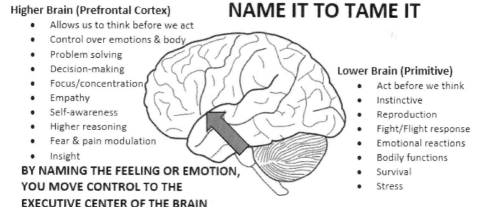

Higher Brain (Prefrontal Cortex)
- Allows us to think before we act
- Control over emotions & body
- Problem solving
- Decision-making
- Focus/concentration
- Empathy
- Self-awareness
- Higher reasoning
- Fear & pain modulation
- Insight

BY NAMING THE FEELING OR EMOTION, YOU MOVE CONTROL TO THE EXECUTIVE CENTER OF THE BRAIN

NAME IT TO TAME IT

Lower Brain (Primitive)
- Act before we think
- Instinctive
- Reproduction
- Fight/Flight response
- Emotional reactions
- Bodily functions
- Survival
- Stress

The moment you start watching your "self-talk", a higher level of consciousness becomes activated. You begin to observe your thoughts and behaviors, and you gain control over your life. It brings to consciousness those emotions, beliefs, and attitudes in our subconscious that are causing our dysfunctional reactions so that we can reprogram our ego defenses to allow us to live a healthy, fulfilling life instead of suffering.

We can control the power to make choices for ourselves about our beliefs and ideals instead of unconsciously reacting to the old programmed reactions. Awareness and awakening to the fact that we have the power to choose is the greatest agent for change. The more you rehearse optimistic thoughts, the more they become habits and ingrained into our nervous system. With time, they will be part of you and you will have made yourself into an altogether different person.

The 2 real world examples below illustrate traffic collision and pain as the stimulus. In that moment of pause between stimulus and response, our thoughts represent our inner voice. Taking the time to monitor and analyze our thoughts and feelings is essential to positive behaviors. Being present in the moment during the pause gives us control and power over our behavior. Stop and acknowledge what you feel: I'm scared, annoyed, afraid, depressed, etc. Always question your "thinking": ask yourself, what is the one thing I can do that could make this better? What is the best response for my happiness and health? Take control over!

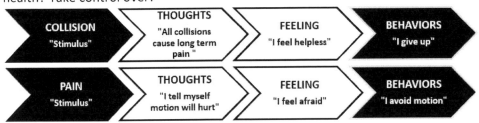

The following are recommendations for chronic pain sufferers:
Way that you think (thoughts, beliefs, emotions, and feelings – our internal voice)

- There are two ways to control your thoughts: You can interrupt and replace them, or you can eliminate them altogether.
- Accurately labeling thoughts, feelings, and emotions can help you cope more effectively. Name it to tame it.
- The basic concept of neuroplasticity is based on the idea that, "neurons that fire together, wire together" and "neurons that fire apart, wire

apart." The great news is that we can rewire our nervous system and reprogram our mental software.

- What you think of yourself is much more important than what others think of you. Love yourself and strive to be the person that you have always wanted to be.
- The way that you think about the future is more important than what happened in the past.
- Monitor your thoughts and beliefs, notice the negative ones, and consciously replace them. Once you get into the habit of disputing negative beliefs, your daily life will run much better and you will feel much happier.
- It is a mistake to "over-think" and make every unwanted aspect of life the symptom of a disorder.
- We are what we think about all day long. Thoughts become things. In other words, "you get what you expect".
- Sustained gratitude is one of the most important states of thought.
- Respond not react (maintain control and power):
- Practice disputing your automatic interpretations of symptoms and events.
- Move thinking to the prefrontal cortex (higher level thinking).
- Watch your thoughts, they become your feelings; watch your feelings, they become your behaviors; watch your behaviors, they become your habits; watch your habits, for it becomes your life.
- We enjoy the benefits of good decisions and pay the consequences for poor decisions.
- If a thought serves you, you keep it. If it doesn't serve you, you reject it.
- The mind is a wonderful servant, but a terrible master.
- Mindfulness is a tool in letting go of the many attachments we often hold on to, such as pain or disability.

The things that you do (actions, response and behavior):
- Behavior is driven by emotions, feelings and thoughts.
- The things that we eat, drink or put into our body have a significant influence on our thoughts, health, and happiness.
- Our body and joints need motion for health and pain relief. Move it or lose it is a fact.
- Strengthening our muscles prevents injury, reduces pain and is essential for health and happiness.
- Sleeping is one of the most important and fundamental aspects of health and happiness.

- Know your limits and avoid things that may exacerbate or relapse your condition.
- Don't take advice from people in worse condition than you are in.
- Laughing when you catch yourself falling back into old negative habits helps you to redirect your mind.
- Let the pain go and focus on health. Attachment to the pain leads to suffering.

The next time you find yourself catastrophizing, anxious, or worried, pause for a moment and pay attention to what you're saying to yourself. We tend to have automatic responses to different situations. We need to develop awareness of those automatic responses and then develop new, more effective ways to interpret life's events. About 80 percent of your worries can be resolved by taking these six steps:

1. Deliberately pause what you're doing and label your feelings and emotions.
2. Writing down precisely what you are worried about or fearful of.
3. Writing down all the things that you can do to make your situation better.
4. Decide the best action to take.
5. Immediately take action with optimism.
6. Reevaluate weekly and modify your plan.

Arête - The best version of you!

Arête is an ancient Greek word that can be best translated as flourishing. Arête is expressing the highest and greatest version of you from moment to moment to moment. The quality of your health and happiness, involves living a good or balanced life. Aristotle stated that everyone should aim to achieve health and happiness in their own lives. Other great teachers have said similar, below is invaluable awareness for you to digest:

Jesus says: "He who rules his spirit has won a greater victory than the taking of a city."

Buddha says: "One who conquers himself is greater than another who conquers a thousand times a thousand men on the battlefield."

Proverbs 4:23 says: "More than anything you guard, protect your mind, for life flows from it."

Jesus says: "Blessed are the tamed and disciplined, for they shall inherit the earth."

Thomas Edison says: "The doctor of the future will give no medicine but will interest his patients in the care of the human frame and in the cause and prevention of disease."

Buddhist proverb says: "Pain is inevitable, suffering is optional."
Benjamin Franklin says: "An ounce of prevention is worth a pound of cure," and "God helps those who help themselves".
William James says: "The greatest discovery of my generation is that human beings can alter their lives by altering their attributes of mind."
Aristotle says: "We are what we repeatedly do. Excellence, then, is not an act, but a habit."
Aristotle also says: "The greatest mistake physicians make is that they attempt to cure the body without attempting to cure the mind; yet the mind and the body are one and should not be treated separately."
C. Norman Shealy, MD says: "Pain is more than a hurt; it is to all too many a way of life."
1 Thessalonians 5:16-18 says: "Rejoice always, pray without ceasing, give thanks in all circumstances".
Eckhart Tolle says: "Nonresistance, nonjudgement, and nonattachment are the three aspects of true freedom & enlightened living."
Deepak Chopra, MD says: "The way you think, the way you behave, and the way you eat can influence your life by 30 to 50 years."
Martin Seligman, PHD says: "Life inflicts the same setbacks and tragedies on the optimist as on the pessimist, but the optimist weathers them better."
Greg McKeown says: "Remember that if you don't prioritize your life, someone else will."
Deepak Chopra says: "A truly wealthy person's attention is never focused on money alone."
FDR says: "Only thing we have to fear is fear itself."
Henry Rollins says: "Sometimes the truth hurts. And sometimes it feels really good."
Pablo Picasso says: "Action is the foundational key to all success."
James Allen says: "You are today where your thoughts have brought you; you will be tomorrow where your thoughts take you."
Ryan Holiday says: "Failure shows us the way – by showing us what isn't the way."
And like Nike says: "Just do it!"

Making health and happiness a habit is Arête. You can also think of this as a rewiring our nervous system and a reprogramming of our mental operating system (software) for health, happiness, and prosperity. The trick is to transform from who you are to whom you're capable of being, so you can enjoy mental and emotional well-being. To make the greatest progress, you don't have to make huge, drastic changes. You just have to take baby steps – but keep on taking them, and don't stop or turn around. Be persistent, and remember. There is no trying, there is only doing!

In Japan, they call this approach kaizen which means continuous improvement. This is a proven long-term approach to improvement that systematically seeks to achieve small, incremental changes in you. It turns out that slow and steady is the best way to overcome your resistance to change. Small and daily micro-wins, when done consistently over time, lead to life-changing habits. It is important to also have long term goals, but daily, small micro-wins equal big wins over time.

BE the person who you would be if you already had achieved health. Then you will DO the things that a healthy person would do, which will allow you to HAVE exactly what you want. **You have to BE healthy before you can BECOME healthy.**

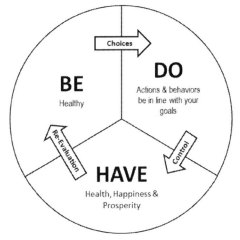

Exercise, motion, flexibility, balance, and strength (the deep spinal stabilizing muscles or deep core muscles) are essential for health. Exercise is good for us mentally, cardiovascularly, metabolically, structurally, as well as most other body systems. Joint motion is essential for joint health, prevents stiffness, and prevents some forms of arthritis. Flexibility helps the ligaments and muscles, as well as joints. Simple balance training helps the nervous system and prevents falls.

Strengthening the deep spinal muscles, specifically the multifidus muscles, is essential for neck and back pain patients. When in doubt, start slow. Remember, no one just wakes up one day and runs a marathon; conditioning takes time and effort. It never hurts to work out a little easier, but working too hard can have adverse consequences. Don't underestimate the therapeutic benefits of walking: it gently stimulates circulation and aerobic muscle fiber activity, is mentally beneficial, and can help redevelop the aerobic system.

Drinking water is the simplest and most effective thing that you can start right away and have big results. It is believed that anywhere up to 75% of Americans spend the vast majority of their time dehydrated and are operating at a deficit as a result. Hydration is critically important to our health, as it helps relieve headaches and stiffness. Water makes up around 75% of our bodies, and it is used in countless crucial functions throughout the body. Water acts as an important catalyst for a number of chemical reactions and forms the basis of everything from neurotransmitters to joint fluid to spinal fluid to our blood.

Make eating healthy a permanent lifestyle and not just a temporary diet. Food is one of the best preventative medicines and an important factor in most chronic diseases. In general, stay away from carbohydrates, sugar and processed foods. About 40 percent of the carbohydrate foods you eat are converted to fat and are inflammatory. Any books by Dr. Mark Hyman, Dr. Daniel Amen, Michael Pollan, Gary Taubes or Dr. Joseph Mercola is a good place to start getting you eating on track.

Sleeping is another simple but essential aspect of health. To understand why sleep is important, think of your body like a factory that performs a number of vital functions. As you drift off to sleep, your body begins its night-shift work: Healing damaged cells, boosting your immune system, recovering from the day's activities, rest your muscles and joints, stress relief, recharging your brain, heart, and cardiovascular system, and much more, so that you can be your best for the next day. Avoid caffeine, computers, phone screens, overstimulation, and TV before bed. A sleep mask, a good mattress, and breathing exercises are wonderful to help with getting restful sleep. Sleep is essential! My top 10 healthy sleep habits:

1. Sleep in a dark, quiet, and cool room. Use a sleep mask.
2. Go "device-free" one hour before bed.
3. Avoid watching TV or reading in bed.
4. Nap wisely (before about 3pm).
5. Get out of bed if you can't sleep; Use 20-minute rule.
6. Maintain a consistent, regular bed time routine.
7. Do not go to bed hungry; go to the bathroom first.
8. Finish exercise 3 hours before bedtime.
9. No alcohol or nicotine 3-6 hours before bed.
10. Stop caffeine 6 hours before bedtime.

Many patients try to do too much too quickly or focus on things not essential to health and happiness. They get frustrated and give up. Greg McKeown makes a compelling case for achieving more by doing less in his great book Essentialism. He reminds us that clarity of focus and the ability to say 'no' to nonessential things are both critical and undervalued. "Essentialism is not about how to get more things done; it's about how to get the right things done. It doesn't mean just doing less for the sake of less either. It is about making the wisest possible investment of your time and energy in order to operate at our highest point of contribution by doing only what is essential." Plain and simple, it's essential for you to be healthy and happy. The best version of you focuses on small, essential, daily micro-wins – kaizen style – to flourish.

Being the best version of you starts with you becoming best friends with and loving yourself. Nobody abuses us more than we abuse ourselves, and that needs to stop ASAP! Stop self-destructive habits and behaviors. Be patient, be persistent, and be kind to yourself. Don Miguel Ruiz says that we must make 5 agreements with ourselves to live with Arête:
The First Agreement: Be Impeccable with Your Word. Speak with integrity.
The Second Agreement: Don't Take Anything Personally.
The Third Agreement: Don't Make Assumptions.
The Fourth Agreement: Always Do Your Best.
The Fifth Agreement: Observe your thoughts, don't believe them automatically. Be skeptical of your thoughts and others' opinions.

Proverbs 4:23-27 tells us: "Be careful what you think, because your thoughts run your life. Don't use your mouth to tell lies; don't ever say things that are not true. Keep your eyes focused on what is right and look straight ahead to what is good. Be careful what you do, and always do what is right. Don't turn off the road of goodness; keep away from evil paths."

Free your mind and flourish
Waronpain.com is a website that I am working on for chronic pain patients. It goes into more detail concerning each anatomical diagnosis and specific treatments. As stated earlier, focusing on flourishing with health, happiness, prosperity, and Arête is more productive than focusing on the pain, but targeted treatments for anatomical pathologies is also essential. Below is a list of my top 30 recommendations to flourish:
1.   You enjoy the benefits of good choices but expect to pay the consequences for bad choices.
2.   Drink ONLY water.

3. Adequate and restful sleep.
4. Move & exercise. Your body and your brain need exercise. Motion is also essential for joint health. If exercise was a pill, you'd be taking just one pill to treat about 10 chronic conditions. Movement can replace many drugs, but no drug can ever replace movement.
5. Food is medicine. Eat good food but not too much, and mostly plants. Burn fat for fuel. Sugar is TOXIC.
6. Fix any structural problems. A good clinical diagnosis and good doctors are essential.
7. Be kind to yourself and others. Love & forgive.
8. Change your habits and change your life. Changing or creating a habit takes at least 3 months.
9. Strengthen your deep spinal stabilizing muscles. Allcore 360, planks, and core-building exercises are essential.
10. Focus on small but essential daily micro-wins, kaizen style.
11. Have clearly defined goals. Have a vision board.
12. Practicing spirituality and arête. Utilize mindfulness and meditation.
13. Let the pain go and do what's needed for health. Pain x (Focus + Attachment + Resistance) = Suffering
14. Be good to your gut. Nurture good intestinal health.
15. Breathe.
16. Keep positive relationships.
17. Enjoy the sun and connect with nature.
18. Live with gratitude.
19. Practice learned optimism and recognize catastrophizing. Expect the best.
20. Move from being Fragile to Resilient to Antifragile.
21. Have good hygiene and posture.
22. "Name it to Tame it". Use your prefrontal cortex. Guard your mind.
23. Be persistent. Don't give up (ever). Fall 7 times, but rise 8 times.
24. Disconnect from social media, video games, drama, and work.
25. Laugh and be happy.
26. Volunteer and serve others.
27. Have a pet.
28. Go to the chiropractor or physical therapist. Get a massage. Go to the spa or sauna.
29. Stay busy and productive. Serve others.
30. Get away or take a vacation.

FURTHER RESOURCES TO SUPPORT THIS CHAPTER

This is just the beginning for your path to flourishing in health and happiness. Always consult with your doctor, but these are additional tools that may help you on your journey:

Optimal living 101 – A great service and wealth of knowledge for you to flourish. Their slogan is, "More wisdom in less time". This is a must!

Allcore360 – Great tool to strengthen the deep core spinal muscles.

Orangetheory Fitness Centers– in 1 hour you get a great combination of exercise, stretching and strengthening.

Bowflex youtube channel – Beginning to advance workouts.

Dr. Joseph Mercola – Great website and books for nutritional and wellness advice.

Dr. Joseph Esposito - Prescription for Extreme Health.

Any works by Nikolai Bogduk, Michele Sterling, William E. Morgan, DC, Sonja Lyubomirsky Ph.D, Deepak Chopra MD, Zig Ziglar, Mark Hyman MD, Daniel Amen MD, Robin A McKenzie MD, Pete Egoscue, Andrew Weil MD, Art Brownstein MD, Dean Ornish, MD, Sunil Pai MD, Jack Challem, Ski Chilton, Conna-Lee Weinberg, Jack Stern MD, Arthur Croft DC, Tony Robins, Oprah, Chris Centeno MD, Martin Seligman Ph.D, Mark P Jensen PhD, Gunter Siegmund MEA, Mike Young, PhD, Eckhart Tolle, Lawrence Nordhoff DC or Robert D. Rondinelli MD, PhD will be helpful in your studies.

DEFINITIONS TO SUPPORT THIS CHAPTER

Self-talk - our inner voice; includes our conscious thoughts as well as our unconscious assumptions or beliefs.

Self - a person's essential being, considered as the object of introspection or reflexive action.

Thoughts - A thought is the process of using your mind to consider or evaluate something. Thought can also refer to the organized beliefs of a period, individual, or group. Observe your thoughts. Don't judge them, observe them. Thinking allows us to make sense of, interpret, represent, or model the world we experience, and to make predictions about our world.

Emotions - Emotion is any conscious experience characterized by intense mental activity and a certain degree of pleasure or displeasure. Emotions originally helped our species survive by producing quick reactions to threat, reward, and everything in between in their environments. Emotional reactions are coded in our genes. The amygdala play a role in emotional arousal and regulate the release of neurotransmitters essential for memory consolidation, which is why emotional memories can be so much stronger and longer-lasting. Emotions precede feelings and are physical and instinctual. Because they are physical, they can be objectively measured by blood flow, brain activity, facial micro-expressions, and body language. Emotion occurs in the following order: cognitive appraisal, physiological changes, and then action.

Feelings - Feelings are the next thing that happens after having an emotion, involve cognitive input, usually subconscious, and cannot be measured precisely. Feelings are best understood as a subjective representation of emotions, private to the individual experiencing them. Feelings are mental experiences of body states, which arise as the brain interprets emotions, themselves physical states arising from the body's responses to external stimuli. (The order of such events is: I am threatened, experience fear, and feel horror.) A feeling is a mental portrayal of what is going on in your body when you have an emotion and is the byproduct of your brain perceiving and assigning meaning to the emotion. Emotions play out in the theater of the body. Feelings play out in the theater of the mind.

Nucleus Accumbens (NAc) - The most widely recognized function is its role in the "reward circuit" of the brain. The nucleus accumbens is an important brain area in forming memories involving prominent environmental stimuli, both positive and negative. These memory stores can be called upon in the future to help us remember how to realize the pleasurable experiences again or how to avoid the aversive ones. The nucleus accumbens predicts the arousal for imminent pain. Therefore, in contrast to somatosensory pathways, which reflect sensory properties of acute noxious stimuli, NAc activity anticipates its analgesic potential on chronic pain. The NAc plays an important role in reward, laughter, pleasure, addiction, fear, and the placebo & nocebo effect. the nucleus accumbens is involved in responses to all motivationally-relevant stimuli, whether rewarding or negative.

Amygdala - (triggers emotions particularly fear) The amygdala is a limbic system structure that is involved in many of our emotions and motivations, particularly those that are related to survival. It is involved in the processing of emotions such as fear, anger, and pleasure. The amygdala is also responsible for determining what memories are stored and where the memories are stored in the brain. During persistent pain states a long-lasting functional plasticity of Amygdala activity contributes to an enhancement of the pain experience, including hyperalgesia, aversive behavioral reactions and affective anxiety-like states.

Prefrontal Cortex - (Thinking part of the brain) The "executive center" of the brain. The prefrontal cortex calms the amygdala, helping us regulate our emotions. Executive function relates to abilities to differentiate among conflicting thoughts, determine good and bad, better and best, same and different, future consequences of current activities, working toward a defined goal, prediction of outcomes, expectation based on actions, and self "control".

Brain studies that show how this naming process can activate the prefrontal cortex and calm the primitive limbic amygdala.

"Name it to tame it" - Simply naming an emotion moves your thought from the primitive limbic system part of your brain (Amygdala) to your prefrontal cortex part of the brain which is the executive center of the brain. The primitive part of the brain can put you into fight or flight mode while the more advanced prefrontal cortex better rationalizes the pain or events. When you "Name it", you actually activate competing brain circuits to the fight or flight & anxiety loops, so it will instantly take the edge off of your feelings of stress, fear or anxiety.

Hebb's Law - Neurons that fire together wire together. Our brain cells communicate with one another through synaptic transmission, one brain cell releases a chemical (neurotransmitter) that engages the next brain cell. This communication process is known as "neuronal firing." When brain cells communicate frequently, the connection between them strengthens. Messages that travel the same pathway in the brain over & over begin to transmit faster & faster. With enough repetition, they become automatic. That's why we can go on automatic pilot with certain functions such as driving home from work or hitting a baseball.

Synaptic Pruning - "Use it or lose it!" Synaptic pruning is thought to be the brain's way of removing connections in the brain that are no longer needed.

Phobia - an extreme or irrational fear of or aversion to something.

Thrive - to prosper or flourish.

Joy - the emotion of great delight or happiness caused by something exceptionally good or satisfying.

Flourish - to grow or develop in a healthy or vigorous way, especially as the result of a particularly favorable environment.

Meme - an idea, behavior, or style that spreads from person to person within a culture, often with the aim of conveying a particular phenomenon, theme, or meaning represented by the meme. A meme acts as a unit for carrying cultural ideas, symbols, or practices that can be transmitted from one mind to another through writing, speech, gestures, rituals, or other imitable phenomena with a mimicked theme.

Ego - A lens made of mental conditioning, through which we see and act on the world. Most people are so completely identified with the voice in the head because of the incessant stream of involuntary and compulsive thinking and the emotions that accompany it. Ego is a dysfunctional relationship with the present moment. The central core of all your mind activity consists of certain repetitive and persistent thoughts, emotions, and reactive patterns that you most strongly identify with, resulting in your self-identity.

Kaizen - continuous improvement.

Self-Discipline - the ability to control one's feelings and overcome one's weaknesses; the ability to pursue what one thinks is right despite temptations to abandon it.

Cognition - the mental action or process of acquiring knowledge and understanding through thought, experience, and the senses. It encompasses processes such as attention, the formation of knowledge, memory and working memory, judgment and evaluation, reasoning and "computation," problem solving and decision making, comprehension, and production of language.

Metacognition - "cognition about cognition," "thinking about thinking," "knowing about knowing," becoming "aware of one's awareness," and higher-order thinking skills. Metacognition refers to a level of thinking that involves active control over the process of thinking that is used in learning situations.

Unconscious incompetence - The individual does not understand or know how to do something and does not necessarily recognize the deficit. They may deny the usefulness of the skill. The individual must recognize their own incompetence and the value of the new skill before moving on to the next stage.

Conscious incompetence - Though the individual does not understand or know how to do something, they recognize the deficit, as well as the value of a new skill in addressing the deficit. The making of mistakes can be integral to the learning process at this stage.

Conscious competence - The individual understands or knows how to do something. However, demonstrating the skill or knowledge requires concentration. It may be broken down into steps, and there is heavy conscious involvement in executing the new skill.

Unconscious competence - The individual has had so much practice with a skill that it has become "second nature" and can be performed easily. As a result, the skill can be performed while executing another task. Competence is wired within our nervous system and mind, becoming a habit.

CLOSING THOUGHTS

Thank you for reading The Truth About Whiplash: A Guide to Getting Better! The core emphasis of this book is to transfer responsibility for your well-being from external factors (doctors, surgeries, medications, testing, therapy) to an internal factor (you). Of course, there are many situations where external remedies and advice are needed, but the way you think and things you do have a significant bearing on your health. You will find that many of the recommendations in this book are also helpful for other pain-related disorders, including work and sports injuries.

Made in the USA
Columbia, SC
19 February 2019